Anti-Inflammatory Diet Your Pathway to Looking and Feeling 10 Years Younger
By Beran Parry

IMPORTANT INFORMATION

The information provided in this book is designed to provide helpful information on the subjects discussed. This book is not meant to be used, nor should it be used, to diagnose or treat any medical condition. For diagnosis or treatment of any medical problem, consult your own physician. The publisher and author are not responsible for any specific health or allergy needs that may require medical supervision and are not liable for any damages or negative consequences from any treatment, action, application or preparation, o any person reading or following the information in this book. References are provided for informational purposes only and do not constitute endorsement of any websites or other sources. Readers should be aware that the websites listed in this book may change.

Anti-Inflammatory Diet Your Pathway to Looking and Feeling 10 Years Younger
By Beran Parry

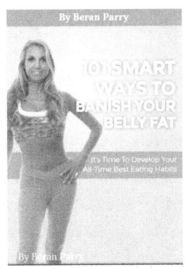

Please search this page over the internet
https://forms.aweber.com/form/14/395417614.htm

Anti-Inflammatory Diet Your Pathway to Looking and Feeling 10 Years Younger
By Beran Parry

WHAT THIS BOOK IS NOT!

Whilst I have referred where appropriate to important medically based studies, books and medical papers, this book has not been written as a medical research paper, designed to cover dozens of scientific subjects.

I have deliberately avoided the current trend in many diet books to constantly cherry pick medical and scientific studies to support the book's conclusions. This book is not intended as a reference item to satisfy those readers that might be looking for useful research material.

There will be a detailed bibliography attached to this book. This is a truly exciting and rapidly evolving science and there is a vast amount of material to read and study about Epigenetics and Functional Medicine in general, especially in the way that these insights apply to intelligent weight management. If you require further information, I suggest you contact me for specific recommendations at beranparry@gmail.com

Anti-Inflammatory Diet Your Pathway to Looking and Feeling 10 Years Younger
By Beran Parry

Copyright © 2017 by Beran Parry

(olw18112017)

All rights reserved. No part of this publication may be reproduced, distributed, or transmitted in any form or by any means, including photocopying, recording, or other electronic or mechanical methods, without the prior written permission of the publisher, except in the case of brief quotations embodied in critical reviews and certain other non-commercial uses permitted by copyright law. For permission requests, write to the author's email address: beranparry@gmail.com

Anti-Inflammatory Diet Your Pathway to Looking and Feeling 10 Years Younger
By Beran Parry

FOR MORE FROM BERAN PARRY

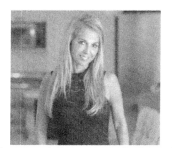

Please search this page over the internet
https://beranparry.com/

Anti-Inflammatory Diet Your Pathway to Looking and Feeling 10 Years Younger
By Beran Parry

Anti-Inflammatory Diet

Your Pathway to

Looking and Feeling

10 Years Younger

By

Beran Parry

Anti-Inflammatory Diet Your Pathway to Looking and Feeling 10 Years Younger
By Beran Parry

Acknowledgements for THIS BOOK.

The inspiration to write this book began more than thirty years ago when I embarked on my first nutritional science courses under the tutelage of Dr Boris Chaitow in South Africa. During the past three decades, I have been most fortunate to receive the guidance, teachings and encouragement of some immensely talented and dedicated doctors and professors. It has been a fascinating journey of exploration, the pathway lit by the giants of natural medicine and naturopathic nutrition. More recently, my studies in the field of Functional Medicine have proved immensely helpful and I would like to pay tribute to the genius, courage and dedication of the following specialists who have assisted me enormously in my quest to share the life-changing knowledge contained in this book.

Among them are Dr Boris Chaitow, Debra Waterhouse, Dr Christiane Northrup, Dr Carolyne Dean, Dr Vasant Lad, Dr Mona Lisa Shulz, Dr Loren Cordain, Dr Patrick Vercammen and Dr Ron Grisanti.

I would particularly like to acknowledge the shining inspiration of a truly remarkable doctor who has been a constant source of knowledge, encouragement and inspiration. Dr Ann Lannoye, a Functional Medicine Specialist and member of the Institute of Functional Medicine, has been a most generous and tireless source of knowledge and enthusiasm for the benefits of Functional Medicine. She provided the inspiration to link my nutritional and eating behaviour work with the Functional Diagnostic Medicine and the analysis of Epigenetic Expression. Dr Lannoye's extensive knowledge and scientific rigour have been one of the major cornerstones of our next book about Functional Medicine in which I hope to have Dr Lannoye join me as a contributor and authority.

My functional medicine research and its conclusions have been so fundamental to my understanding of intelligent nutrition, that I undertook studies at the Functional Medicine University in South Carolina. Dr Ron Grisanti has been a most generous provider of case study information in these vitally important subjects.

I am also delighted to announce a series of further projects with Dr Ann Lannoye and Greg Parry PhD, also based in the field of Functional Medicine. We are scheduling a series of international seminars, professional training courses and wellbeing conventions. If you would like to know more go to... www.beranparry.com

Anti-Inflammatory Diet Your Pathway to Looking and Feeling 10 Years Younger
By Beran Parry

Table of Contents

Chapter 1 13
About Beran 13
Chapter 2: The Definition of Mid-Life Wellbeing Challenges 19
Chapter 3: 21
The 10 YEARS YOUNGER 21
Myth-Buster Chart 21
Chapter 4: 29
So Why Can't I Lose Weight? And why can't I keep the weight off? 29
Create Good Habits 31
Managing your Environment 31
Cravings 32
Addictions. Are you a food junkie? 32
Your Internal Digestion Clock 33
Chapter 5: 37
How You React to Stress and Inflammation Explained 37
How Females deal with Mid Life Challenges 37
Chapter 6: 43
10 YEARS YOUNGER 43
Medical Minimally Invasive Aesthetic Anti-Ageing Procedures 43
Anti-Aging Non-Surgical Treatments Explained 47
Chapter 7: 49
Epigenetics + Long Term Eating Behaviours = Your Present Weight Level 49
The 10 YEARS YOUNGER Three Golden Food Rules! 53
Chapter 8: 59
Introduction to The 10 YEARS YOUNGER Skin Beauty in Midlife 59
Foods that Improve your Appearance from the Inside Out 60
Chapter 9: 63
Getting Organised! 63
Chapter 10: 69
GUT BIOLOGY 69
Chapter 11: 75
YOUR New Career 75
The 10 YEARS YOUNGER Epigenetic Shopping Guide 79
Chapter 12: 89
How Toxins affect weight loss and ageing 89
Chapter 13: 93
The Exercise and 10 YEARS YOUNGER Plan 93
Epigenetic Exercise Myth 93
Chapter 14: 107

Anti-Inflammatory Diet Your Pathway to Looking and Feeling 10 Years Younger
By Beran Parry

Your anti-ageing and weight loss helpers! Vitamin D and Magnesium 107
Chapter 15: 115
10 YEARS YOUNGER DAILY FOOD AND DINING OUT GUIDE 115
Chapter 16: 121
FIFTY 10 YEARS YOUNGER Recipes at your disposal 121
1. Ginger Carrot Protein Smoothie 122
2. Raspberry Coconut Smoothie 123
3. Pineapple Protein Smoothie 124
4. High Protein and Nutritional Delish Smoothie 125
5. Tantalizing Key Lime Pie Smoothie 126
6. Zucchini Fish Soup Delight! 127
7. Roasted Winter Vegetable Turkey Soup 129
8. Turkey Squash Soup 131
9. Delicious Lemon-Garlic Soup 132
10. Creamy Chicken Soup 133
11. Creamy Carrot Salad 135
12. Tasty Carrot Salad 136
13. Asian Aspiration Salad 137
14. Italian Tuna Bonanza Salad 138
15. Incredibly Delish Avocado Tuna Salad 139
16. Avocado and Shrimp Omelette 140
17. Mushrooms, Eggs and Onion Bonanza 142
18. Spectacular Eggie Salsa 143
19. Delish Veggie Hash With Eggs 145
20. Spicy Spinach Bake 146
21. Zucchini Casserole 147
22. Spicy Granola 148
23. Breakfast Mexicana 149
24. Gutsy Granola 151
25. Delish Veggie Breakfast Peppers 152
26. Tasty Apple Almond Coconut Medley 153
27. Sweetie Skinny Crackers 154
28. Apple Chia Delight 155
29. Ultimate Skinny Granola 156
30. Divine Protein Muesli 157
31. Prawn garlic Fried "Rice" 158
32. Delish Baked dill Salmon 160
33. Ostrich Steak or Venison with Divine Mustard Sauce and Roasted Tomatoes 161
34. Scrumptious Cod in Delish Sauce 163
35. Delicious Turkey Veggie Lasagne 164
36. Skinny Veggie Dip 167

Anti-Inflammatory Diet Your Pathway to Looking and Feeling 10 Years Younger
By Beran Parry

37. Delish Cashew Butter Treats 168
38. Chocolate Goji Skinny Bars 169
39. Skinny Power Balls 170
40. Butternut Squash-raw Veggie Dip 172
Chapter 17: 173
The Growing Young Disgracefully Vision 173
Before You Go 178
Bibliography 182

Anti-Inflammatory Diet Your Pathway to Looking and Feeling 10 Years Younger
By Beran Parry

Anti-Inflammatory Diet Your Pathway to Looking and Feeling 10 Years Younger
By Beran Parry

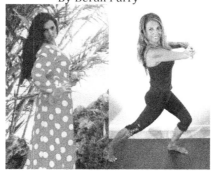

BEFORE   AFTER

My Story

Chapter 1

About Beran

As a Bestselling Diet, Nutrition and Fitness Author, with over 20 bestselling Amazon Books to her credit, Beran Parry is passionate about helping YOU permanently improve YOUR Midlife Health, Weight and Wellbeing!

She is fully Certified (Distinction) in Nutritional Therapy, Advanced Diet and Weight Loss, Exercise Physiology and a Pilates Master Teacher.

After helping thousands of women with their Midlife weight and wellbeing challenges, she can to help YOU transform your life forever!

Beran has also trained over 100 Pilates Teachers Worldwide, she is also a Face Pilates Specialist, a Yoga Teacher and has studied with the Top Functional Medicine Doctor in Europe.

Beran's Story

I am a Thyroid Cancer Survivor. I have had a Subtotal Thyroidectomy and been taking synthetic thyroid hormone for over 17 years. I have gained and lost 50 pounds 3 times in my life!

Anti-Inflammatory Diet Your Pathway to Looking and Feeling 10 Years Younger
By Beran Parry

Despite a slow Metabolism, I lost almost 20 pounds during the midlife transition to menopause by simply following my own detailed and precisely targeted research process, a program that has resulted in a complete transformation of my energy levels, my weight, my body shape, my mental and emotional wellbeing and my ability to fully engage and enjoy life!

I had the worst time ever 18 years ago…..

In 1999, I had the worst year ever when my mother needed emergency lifesaving open heart surgery, I discovered a thyroid malignancy, I also had major personal relationship challenges and a miscarriage due to non-functioning thyroid and hormone imbalance issues!

Imagine a year where your mother is seriously ill, you get a malignancy diagnosis, you suffer a miscarriage, your marriage is in crisis and you hate your work so much that you feel ill just going to the office every day! That happened to me! The year before I thought everything was wonderful! Fabulous marriage, successful career in finance, although I was having low thyroid symptoms and not realizing it!

A huge feeling of despondency and depression descended on me. I now understand fully what its like to feel utterly devastated with life at every level, my health, my weight, my family's health, my marriage, my job and my emotional framework

Fast forward to 2000 and I really had to sit down and take stock of my life, undergo thyroid removal surgery, deal with low metabolism symptoms, patch up the marriage and admit that my office work was affecting my health!

In 2001, I decided to change my life completely, went back to school to restudy Nutrition, Professional Fitness, Pilates, Yoga and Holistic Therapies and I became a Pilates and Reiki Master.

2002-2012

Things went reasonably well during this period of intense study, research and consulting, but I never quite got to the peak health I wanted, because there were clearly post menopausal issues as well as functional medical issues with inflammatory processes in my gut! and I ended up with quite sensational health challenges post menopause in 2013!

In the past, I suffered from irritable bowel syndrome and in 2013 I had a major healing crisis which affected my nervous system and I was unable to work for 6 months. It became the most challenging yet most exciting educational experience of my life as I discovered functional medicine and created a new eating and supplement plan that healed all my inflammation and nervous system symptoms.

Anti-Inflammatory Diet Your Pathway to Looking and Feeling 10 Years Younger
By Beran Parry

The reason this REALLY excited me was because during my research I discovered through functional medicine that my new way of eating had already helped SO MANY ILL PEOPLE with so many challenging conditions besides obesity. These included auto immune issues, cardio vascular issues, malignancies, hormonal issues, and SO MUCH MORE!

Now I am physically and mentally stronger than I was in my 20's, 30's and 40's

My life has been full of challenges and learning experiences on many levels: personally, professionally, through menopause and through many emotional challenges and spiritual quests...... but it has ALL made me SO MUCH STRONGER THAN I EVER WAS!

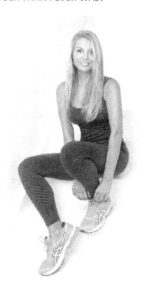

Anti-Inflammatory Diet Your Pathway to Looking and Feeling 10 Years Younger
By Beran Parry

My One Major Reoccurring Challenge

I gained over 50 lbs three times in my life during divorce, pregnancy and trans-Atlantic house moves and each time I recovered and lost even more weight to end up at 10 pounds below my teenage weight for the last 10 years!!! During these intense learning experiences, I discovered SO MANY INTERESTING ways I can help you with your quest for excellent wellbeing!

I now live with my best ever body shape, eat a varied, delicious and plentiful diet, exercise and meditate joyously each day and love my life with passion, peace, energy and joy.

I believe that YOU TOO can live YOUR LIFE with passion, peace, energy and joy!

We are going to work together to change behaviors and MAKE THIS HAPPEN FOR YOU!

My passion in life is to dedicate myself to facilitating this same kind of change in anyone who has been through health challenges, particularly around midlife, and I love to inspire real and permanent change and transformation within every person that I work with. It's my raison d'etre

Now, I specialize in helping anyone with Midlife Health and Weight Issues to achieve their personal life and health goals through mindset, habits, exercise and nutritional programs based on functional medicine concepts.

I always advocate holistic wellbeing, healthy lifestyles, the safest and most effective ways for sustained weight loss, Pilates, yoga and body weight training and paleo/keto nutrition.

Daily, I lecture, consult and coach all over the world via skype and in person to empower others to achieve their lifelong health ambitions and turn their goals and dreams into reality

I also run Ultimate Midlife Detox and Boot Camp Retreats around the world to get YOUR Body and Health into its BEST SHAPE EVER!

Now I am dedicating my life and knowledge to help you create YOUR very BEST Wellbeing and Weight Loss Programs

Beran Parry is passionate about helping people around the world reach their wellbeing, fitness, health and weight loss goals;

She is a certified and specialized Nutritional therapist and Advanced Diet and Weight Loss Consultant. She also holds certifications in Exercise Physiology, Pilates, Reiki and EFT.

Anti-Inflammatory Diet Your Pathway to Looking and Feeling 10 Years Younger
By Beran Parry

Beran is also a Master Pilates Trainer, a face Pilates specialist and yoga teacher and a meditation and EFT therapist.

Beran resides in Spain but constantly travels to the USA, UK, Belgium, South Africa and Germany to lecture, consult and lead wellbeing retreats for an international audience. She also consults via skype, telephone, email, video chats and at her local facilities.

Anti-Inflammatory Diet Your Pathway to Looking and Feeling 10 Years Younger
By Beran Parry

As a special seasonal gift I would like to offer you my 5 day Paleo Detox at a 50% discount to do before or after the Holiday Season. It contains the following exciting elements

Delicious Recipes,

Stunning Detox Menu's,

Detoxifying Pilates Exercise Videos,

A Daily Detox Face Pilates Program,

Guided Detox Meditations,

FREE Bonus Recipe Books,

FREE Stress Release System

Here is more info and the coupon code

beranparry.com/midlife-fatburn-detox

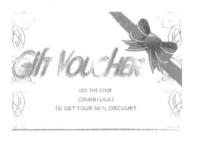

Anti-Inflammatory Diet Your Pathway to Looking and Feeling 10 Years Younger
By Beran Parry

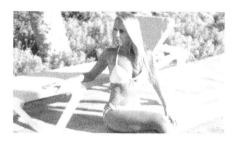

Chapter 2: The Definition of Mid-Life Wellbeing Challenges

10 YEARS YOUNGER means courageous living. It means establishing a new relationship to time, where you stop fearing it or trying to outrun it because, when you're living agelessly, you don't pay attention to your age, whatever it is.

If you aren't thinking about how old you are at the moment, then a milestone birthday or a lifestyle-related illness of someone close might make you reflect on how you could change your lifestyle and get older without deteriorating. Many women suddenly develop an auto-immune disorder, a pre-cancerous or cancerous condition, or allergies. If it's not a health crisis that's thrown them off course, it's the loss of a partner, a career choice or a dependable person or situation.

Why do women and men resign themselves to the negative effects and potential pitfalls of aging? Is it simply because we prefer to hand over the responsibility for our health to a person in a white coat? Or is it because we don't believe we are capable of making our own mid-life wellbeing decisions for our own bodies. Experiencing the symptoms of aging can be scary, but why not place some trust in our own ability to recognise what we need to do? Of course we need to educate ourselves to be able to make informed decisions and that's exactly what I want to help you to do.

I want to help you to learn about what is happening to your body and about what natural choices are available to assist you through this process of change. A change that can really be for the better if you allow yourself this experience.

It's so tempting to hand over responsibility for how you want to feel to a medical professional who does not necessarily know what it feels like to be you. How on earth can they?

Anti-Inflammatory Diet Your Pathway to Looking and Feeling 10 Years Younger
By Beran Parry

In my holistic wellness practise, I have met up with thousands of woman going through aging challenges, women from age 35 all the way up to 90, and it's been a startling revelation to learn about the attitude of resignation that exists about the negative effects of aging and its associated health challenges

Through a lack of awareness of the many safe choices that exist for us, woman have tended to disregard that nature itself has its own wisdom about these matters and working with nature using natural alternatives can produce and recreate radiant good health throughout the entire midlife period and way beyond.

Growing older is an opportunity for you to increase your value and competence as the neural connections throughout your brain increase, weaving into your brain and body the wisdom of a life well lived, which allows you to stop living out of fear of disappointing others and being imperfect. (see references at end of chapter)

So here you are, at an intersection, where you have to make a decision about what your lifestyle and your life will be like in the years to come. The fact that you are reading this right now is absolute proof that you are really ready for absolute improvement in some or all areas of your life! If you weren't seriously thinking about changing your approach to your life, you wouldn't be here with me right now.

So are you going to grow older with guts or degenerate with age? Will you stick with battling the body to get it to behave itself? Will you continue putting other people's requirements ahead of your own and will you keep fuelling yourself with processed foods, sugar, caffeine, anxiety, and stress? Or will you get off the path that leads to illness, frailty, and reduced quality of life and start living with courage and vitality, as if you really mean it?

of your own destiny. Forget about waiting around for someone else to arrive and make your dreams come true. *You* must make your own happiness and pleasure a priority.

At first, that might sound a bit crazy and even selfish. It certainly bucks convention, doesn't it? But when you realize beyond a shadow of a doubt that you're not only *able* to create your own pleasure, but that you're also *responsible* for it, you'll stop being disappointed in (and angry with) other people who either can't or won't do it for you. This doesn't mean that no one else can bring you joy and pleasure. They certainly can! But when you take responsibility for giving yourself what you want and need (as well as making requests of others, when appropriate), you'll feel more in control of your life and less like a victim at the mercy of the whims of others. Taking this step is deliciously empowering!

(Areas of this chapter adapted from the book Ageless Goddess by Northrup, Dr C)

Anti-Inflammatory Diet Your Pathway to Looking and Feeling 10 Years Younger
By Beran Parry

Chapter 3:

The 10 YEARS YOUNGER

Myth-Buster Chart

The Epigenetic Myth-Buster Chart - your 5 point blueprint and lifelong passport to the happy realm of total weight control and permanent residence in the Land of Fitter and Skinnier.

CMR Conventional Medical Recommendation.

DEFINITION: The old view of what is supposed to be good for you.

SPS Skinny Paradigm Shift.

DEFINITION: The revolutionary new advances in medical and scientific research that will transform your health

Let's get serious. Fact: If the old ways worked, we wouldn't be having an explosion of obesity in the developed world and we wouldn't be having this conversation, would we? Clearly something is missing. Our mission is to show you what the problem really is, how to fix the problem and fix it forever.

Anti-Inflammatory Diet Your Pathway to Looking and Feeling 10 Years Younger
By Beran Parry

Steps	CMR	SPS
1. Grains	Insists that grains are actually good for you. Wheat, rice, corn, cereal, bread, pasta etc. Most governments recommend 8-10 servings per day as the principle daily source of energy, nutrition and fibre. Entire industries are devoted to promoting this idea as the healthiest way to live. Ask pretty much anyone and they'll tell you how good it is to eat grains.	UCLA lecturer and world famous evolutionary biologist Jared Diamond stipulates 'Grains are the worst mistake of the human race.' In nutritional terms, grains are simply inferior to plants. Grains trigger insulin production and fat storage. They produce allergic reactions, suppress the immune response and trigger a wide range of intolerances as well as imbalances in the intestinal flora.
2. Fats	Fat makes you fat therefore if you reduce fat you'll lose fat. The world is awash with countless 'fat free' and 'low fat' products and we have a ballooning obesity problem.	Good quality fat drives efficient fat and protein metabolism, encouraging weight loss and boosting energy levels.
3. Meal Habits	Three square meals a day plus snacks are best to stave off hunger pangs and stabilise metabolism	Any steps to normalise your insulin production encourages your skinny genes to take over. Occasional fasting using protein soup meals can help you to reprogram your fat burning potential
4. Cardio exercise	30-60 minutes cardio per day. Lift weights regularly using isolated parts of the body and aim for maximum resistance, even going for the point of failure to increase strength.	Weight resistance using the whole body in short bursts plus slower more regular cardio exercise for shorter periods per day with sporadic intense bursts of intensity. This system really does work!

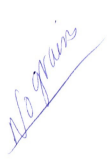

Anti-Inflammatory Diet Your Pathway to Looking and Feeling 10 Years Younger
By Beran Parry

Steps	CMR	SPS
5. sun exposure	Wear sunscreen every day, in all weather and in every season. It should have a sun protection factor (SPF) of 30 and say "broad-spectrum" on the label, which means it protects against the sun's UVA and UVB rays. Put it on at least 15 minutes before going outside. Use 1 ounce, which would fill a shot glass	Sunshine can be a tricky thing. We need it, but it can also be harmful. Striking the right balance between getting enough sunshine to produce optimal levels of Vitamin D, and protecting ourselves from the harm the sun can do, can be a challenge. Most experts recommend 15-20 minutes of sun exposure several times a week for the average fair-skinned person, as this is enough to produce optimal levels of Vitamin D while not being so much to damage skin. Darker skin tones with more melanin need to stay in the sun longer to synthesize vitamin D effectively...see more info below Vitamin D, which our body produces when we are exposed to sunlight, does wonders for us - from improving mood to boosting our immune systems, reducing inflammation and much more, it's key to our health. According to some new research, it seems there is yet another reason to get the right amount of sunlight. Researchers found that older women (65+) with low Vitamin D levels are more likely to gain weight.

(see references at end of chapter)

Time Bomb Triggers

It's very controversial but it looks increasingly likely that humans made a massive and deeply influential error around seven thousand years ago. It wasn't intended as an error. It happened because

Anti-Inflammatory Diet Your Pathway to Looking and Feeling 10 Years Younger
By Beran Parry

it looked exactly like a brilliant strategy for survival. In fact the idea was so good that it rapidly spread and became the foundation for human civilisation. The brilliant idea was agriculture.

Brilliant because it helped to solve the constant challenge of ensuring a regular food supply. A profound error because it encouraged our ancestors to become completely dependent on grains. Seven thousand years ago is effectively yesterday in evolutionary terms. Our bodies did not evolve to exist on a grain-rich diet. But that is what has happened over the last seven thousand years.

The human genome hasn't changed very much during this time span but our diet and lifestyle have diverged dramatically from the way our ancestors lived before the introduction of agriculture. It is believed that many of our contemporary diseases have arisen as a result of this revolution in our dietary habits.

We'll take a closer look at these important issues as we explore the great behaviours you can use to transform your weight and your life. For now let's concentrate on the more obvious consequences of the way we eat.

You've probably already guessed the most obvious outcome of these changes in our diet; an astonishing increase in disease at a time of unprecedented medical advances. Scientists are beginning to suspect a common cause to this tendency towards disease: it's all in our diet. Seven thousand years might not have been long enough for humans to have adapted successfully to a grain-oriented diet. And then, of course, we have the strange phenomenon of obesity. The problem, like many waistlines, is getting bigger.

In 1980 there were approximately 875 million overweight and obese people in the world. In 2013, the number had grown to 2.1 billion. That's an increase of 28% in adult obesity and, more alarmingly, a 47% increase in the number of overweight children in just the past thirty-three years. What could be causing such a radical shift in the average size and weight of humans in such a dramatically short period of time? The answer might lie within us. Or, to be more precise, within our gut.

Recent discoveries about the trillions of microorganisms that live in and on the human body are now changing the traditional perspective on human health and disease. In terms of obesity, we're learning that it's not just heredity and gene expression related to our human genome that play a role, but also the trillions of microorganisms that make up the vastly larger (in terms of unique genetic material) second genome in our body, the human microbiome. Studies have begun to describe each human gut as a highly complex eco-system, populated by communities of bacteria as well by viruses, fungi and moulds. The contents of our gut seem to exert an extraordinary influence on our digestive system, but these micro flora also affect our health in general, our wellbeing and even our mental and emotional balance. Imbalances in the micro flora of the gut have now been identified as an important

Anti-Inflammatory Diet Your Pathway to Looking and Feeling 10 Years Younger
By Beran Parry

cause of obesity. The gut's microbiome, that miniature universe within our digestive system, is where many of our health and weight issues are focused.

The obese gut microcosm

One of the disorders that we now know is associated with an altered gut microflora is obesity. There is a wealth of fascinating evidence from initial studies that reveal a distinct connection between the microbes in our gut and the way our bodies regulate fat storage. These results have been widely replicated and numerous other reports have confirmed this relationship. By now it's well established that obesity is characterised by an obese-oriented microbiota and that gut microbes really can influence fat storage through a variety of mechanisms.

Adding depth to our understanding of the obesity problem, we know that obesity is virtually unheard of in hunter-gatherer populations and the same observation holds true for many non-westernised societies. So we can conclude that obesity is predominantly a disease of civilised, grain-consuming societies. There's a major clue here about some of the causes of unhealthy weight gain that dominate developed societies.

We can look a little deeper into this question about the influence of our gut flora. Obese or overweight people have different gut flora compared to lean individuals. Yes they do. Hunter gatherers also have a very different microbiome compared to the intestinal flora of westernised peoples. And we know that hunter gatherers don't do fat! It also seems clear that flora in the gut can influence metabolic hormones such as leptin and insulin, key influencers in the body's inflammatory response. Research is identifying the extraordinary role of prebiotics, probiotics and other microbiome stabilisers in encouraging fat loss in humans and animals. Surprised? Utterly amazed that changing and re-balancing your gut flora can be so beneficial for your health and weight loss issues? Stay with me, my friend. We're just getting started!

More on the importance of correct sun exposure.

Vitamin D, which our body produces when we are exposed to sunlight, does wonders for us – from improving mood to boosting our immune systems, reducing inflammation and much more, it's key to our health. According to some new research, it seems there is yet another reason to get the right amount of sunlight. Researchers found that older women (65+) with low Vitamin D levels are more likely to gain weight

Folks, without question, the best way to get the right amount of vitamin D is to spend some time in the sun.

Anti-Inflammatory Diet Your Pathway to Looking and Feeling 10 Years Younger
By Beran Parry

You always want to avoid getting burned, but generally speaking you can safely spend anywhere from 20 minutes to two hours in the sun every day with beneficial effects. If you have dark-colored skin or live far from the equator, you will need to spend more time in the sun than someone who is light-skinned living close to the equator.

There are many available books and studies on the benefits and risks of too sunlight and vitamin d depletion. Contact me for a recommend reading list at beranparry@gmail.com

It's becoming clear now that the pathway to sustainable health and wellbeing, to a leaner, fitter, stronger and happier body is not in the outdated Conventional Medical Recommendations. The future is in the Epigenetics Revolution and the Epigenetic Paradigm Shift.

Soma areas of this chapter adapted from the book Primal Blueprint (Sisson, M)

Anti-Inflammatory Diet Your Pathway to Looking and Feeling 10 Years Younger
By Beran Parry

Summary – Myth buster

The folly of grains in the human diet

Welcome to the inner universe of your microbiome

Being overweight is closely connected to the state of your gut flora

CMR versus SPS

SPS - The smarter way to live long, lose weight and live better

Anti-Inflammatory Diet Your Pathway to Looking and Feeling 10 Years Younger
By Beran Parry

Anti-Inflammatory Diet Your Pathway to Looking and Feeling 10 Years Younger By Beran Parry

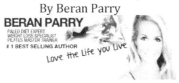

Chapter 4:

So Why Can't I Lose Weight? And why can't I keep the weight off?

These are good questions because even champion weight losers often put the weight back on, suffering the seemingly inevitable see-saw effect of cyclical weight loss followed by weight gain. Can we do something to correct this problem? Of course we can! That's exactly what this book is for.

SKINNY PARADIGM PYRAMID 1 – YOUR BIGGEST WEIGHT INFLUENCER

Anti-Inflammatory Diet Your Pathway to Looking and Feeling 10 Years Younger
By Beran Parry

YOUR GENETICS - 10%
Genes can be outsmarted by epigenetics
Your Gut holds the Secrets of Healthy Weightloss

YOUR FOOD SELECTION PROCESS – 30%
What and When YOU Eat Makes the Difference
Your Food Choices are the Critical Factor
Your Challenge is to really Learn how to Eat Smart, Eat Right and Feel Great

YOUR EATING BEHAVIOUR – 60%
Eating Behaviour Rules the Scales
Personal Choices Always Produce Inevitable Consequences
Choosing the Right Priorities when it comes to What and How and When we Eat,
Time Management when it relates to your Eating Behaviour can be your biggest Friend or Enemy

As you might recall from my life story, over the years of battling with weight issues, I tried many, many different methods and diets to lose weight and keep the pounds off. In those early years, with very little useful help or advice, I experienced most of the recurring problems that I bet you're familiar with. Every "weight loss program" was slow and the weight certainly didn't come off very quickly. This was always frustrating and de-motivating. With the SPS weight loss protocol this problem is solved. I lost a total of fifty pounds over the course of eighteen months. When you are losing weight gradually but consistently every day, this keeps your motivation at a very high level. The next problem with every other weight loss system I tried is that I was always hungry and that made me feel pretty miserable most of the time. Does that sound familiar to you? Clearly a better way is needed!

Anti-Inflammatory Diet Your Pathway to Looking and Feeling 10 Years Younger
By Beran Parry

Create Good Habits

Willpower - the mantra of the naturally thin. Why willpower alone is overrated

Let's just accept that we're going to need more than willpower to get the job done. When you rely on willpower alone you set yourself up for failure and disappointment. Routine and old habits are strongly embedded in our behaviour so they will win out over willpower 99% of the time and this is another reason why diets simply don't work. They rely on short-term changes that no normal person can ever hope to maintain.

A good habit doesn't require willpower or discipline. By definition, a habit is something you don't even think about. It's something that you do or feel automatically. Bad habits don't usually take up too much of your attention either until you begin to suffer the consequences. Because bad habits inevitably have a down side. If there's a habit you're trying to change, you need to be motivated to do something about it. Most of us respond positively to a suitable reward (not food!) to make the change worthwhile and repeatable.

You need a simple structure to help you modify your behaviour in the simplest way possible. And you need a starting point. This can be anything from a personal coach, a good friend or colleague who will keep reminding you or even family members to encourage you. It only takes 3 weeks to internalise your new behaviour and make it a permanent and positive habit that can last a lifetime. And the absolute perfect time to start is right now. In the next few chapters we are going to show you how.

Managing your Environment

Before we take a closer look at the mechanics of smart weight loss, we need to think about how we can boost our chances of success by monitoring our environment. You don't have to be a certified Boy or Girl Scout but *Being Prepared* can help you anticipate potential problems when temptation is likely to roll across your path. If you know you're going to be in a situation where the wrong food is likely to be available, you can avoid the problems by preparing yourself in advance. This is something I do automatically these days. I'll take my own food along when I go out with friends or ask for a meal that fits my dietary requirements. It's that easy. You are psychologically so much better prepared to resist all the garbage that passes for typical hotel or restaurant catering that you won't even notice all the usual no-go areas. And you will feel so much better because you've respected your body's natural nutrition needs. Keep the garbage food out of your home, away from the work place and out of your life. Don't torture yourself by stocking up on things that are killing you and then struggling to resist them. Make everything so much easier by keeping all the bad stuff out of sight. The longer you stay on the right track, the more your body will detox and the easier it will feel for you to do the right thing effortlessly all the time.

Anti-Inflammatory Diet Your Pathway to Looking and Feeling 10 Years Younger
By Beran Parry

Cravings

Intense hunger. Thin people can never understand this. It's a hard but inescapable fact. An overweight person is physically hungry more often than a naturally thin person. And the hunger is much more intense. Thin people frequently accuse overweight people of lacking the self-control to stop eating. It's a great story and it makes thin people feel better. But it is absolutely not true. Not. True. The thin person cannot possibly comprehend the intense physiological and almost constant hunger that overweight people have to deal with. It has nothing to do with self-control. This is a real, gnawing, overwhelming and intense physical hunger. That's a good reason why those very fortunate, naturally thin people and exercise gurus should not write books on how to lose weight. They have no concept of the scale and depth of the challenges that overweight people have to deal with on a daily basis. You have to know what those hunger drives really feel like before you start giving advice! One of the startling revelations that we're going to explore together is the fact that many overweight people are starving. Their bodies are starved of essential nutrients so they're constantly hungry and their bodies are crying out for something nutritiously worthwhile to satisfy those basic needs. It's so ironic that obese individuals feel so hungry but it's a reality that we're going to deal with by fixing the problem right at its source.

Eating when your body doesn't need the fuel.

Overweight people are also prone to problems with "emotional eating" or cravings. Certain food cravings fall into the above hunger category as they are certainly physiological in nature. Other food cravings or emotional eating occur when you are physically not hungry, but your hunger becomes a displacement activity to satisfy unfulfilled emotional needs. This hunger might be emotional in origin but it feels exactly like real physical hunger when you experience it.

Addictions. Are you a food junkie?

During the 1980s when the arrival of highly processed, cheap cocaine in the form of crack produced an epidemic in drug addiction, researchers were convinced that of all the substances that could cause addiction in humans, food simply could not be classed as addictive. Scientists absolutely refused to consider the possibility that an individual could become addicted to any kind of food. It just wasn't possible.

Over-eating was considered to be a behavioural problem that could be fixed with a little self-discipline, a treadmill and some much needed self-control. But during the 1990s, as obesity rates soared, researchers began to apply brain-scanning technology to investigate what really happened in the brains of obese people. The results were astonishing. Overweight people displayed the same chemical reactions to food that had been detected in drug addicts. Obese people were showing signs of real, measurable, chemical addiction to food. And the addiction usually applied to the unhealthiest food possible.

In fact, as weight management specialists began to record their patients' attitudes and behaviour in thousands of detailed reports, it became clear that vast numbers of overweight people were struggling with a powerful, irresistible addiction to the worst kinds of foodstuffs. The problem is linked to the brain's reward system and the powerful chemical, dopamine. As individuals receive overwhelming bursts of pleasure and satisfaction from their food intake, the brain switches off dopamine receptors to reduce the effect of the pleasure rush. So the body needs more raw fuel in the form of the pleasure-inducing, comforting foods to achieve the same levels of satisfaction. It's a vicious circle and then it gets worse.

The change in brain chemistry erodes the link with the Pre-Frontal Cortex, the adult part of the brain that can exercise control over excessive behaviour. So we lose contact with the part of the brain that can regulate our addiction and the situation gets out of hand. The result is obesity and all the health problems that go along with it.

So it really is important to recognise the addictive nature of food and understand that we will need to train our behaviour to find other, healthier ways to get our dopamine rush. For most people, a wake-up call is usually the moment of realisation that something really has to change. A wake-up call that can sometimes be scary but motivates us to make changes in our behaviour and tackle the addiction.

Your Internal Digestion Clock

Eating too late in the evening is a disaster for good digestion and for good sleep. Food and alcohol can disrupt the body's natural digestive cycles and encourage the body to store the food as fat. There's a great deal of interesting modern research on this fascinating topic but the concept is hardly new.

When we consider the health issues of eating too late in the day, one of the unfortunate side effects of bingeing close to bedtime is an increase in blood sugar levels for a full 24 hours. This conclusion was published in a study in *Obesity Research & Clinical Practice*.

Meanwhile, research in the *Journal of Clinical Sleep Medicine* confirms that eating high-calorie, high-fat snacks at night results in restless sleep. This can result in overeating the next day in an attempt to boost flagging energy levels.

Anti-Inflammatory Diet Your Pathway to Looking and Feeling 10 Years Younger
By Beran Parry

As a general rule of thumb, experts now suggest eating 90 percent of your total calories during the day, focusing on lunch as the main meal of the day. That still leaves you a healthy 150 to 200 calories to consume in a 'smart snack' before you go to bed.

Genetics.

There are thousands of diet books, countless weight-loss articles and hundreds of weight loss organisations but we all know about the real problem of losing weight; the fat begins to slip away, we post the good news on Facebook, celebrating the success - and then we see all the good work undone as we put the pounds back on in a very short period of time. Now that is just too frustrating!

Relax. Help is finally at hand. We'll show how to re-set your metabolism and take control of your weight issues for the rest of your life.

If you still suspect that your inherited DNA is responsible for making you overweight, I'd like to repeat that it's being proved time and time again that genetics simply do not play the only role in causing obesity. Genetics can be thanked for your general body shape but are not the main cause for a low metabolism, intense and constant physical hunger, or emotional eating. The answer lies in our behaviour and in our environment. In other words, our weight is entirely a product of what we do.

Do things differently and the weight ceases to be problem.

Excited? Stay with me. Read on! We're just getting started!

Anti-Inflammatory Diet Your Pathway to Looking and Feeling 10 Years Younger
By Beran Parry

SUMMARY

Metabolism is the key

Recognising intense hunger and cravings

Creating good habits

Managing your environment

Building support from friends, family and colleagues

Eliminating the villains from the weight loss narrative

Anti-Inflammatory Diet Your Pathway to Looking and Feeling 10 Years Younger
By Beran Parry

Anti-Inflammatory Diet Your Pathway to Looking and Feeling 10 Years Younger
By Beran Parry

Chapter 5:

How You React to Stress and Inflammation Explained

The subject of stress can be quite confusing. It's such a pervasive facet of our lives that it's easy to mistake it for a natural phenomenon. But it isn't. It's time to add a measure of much-needed clarity to the subject. It is essential that we do not mistake the events around us as being the source of our stress. They are simply events. Nothing more and nothing less.

It's our conditioned reflex to our external and internal landscapes that determines whether or not we trigger the stress response. Most of us are heavily conditioned from early childhood to feel stressed under a wide variety of circumstances. Just because virtually everyone is blighted by the effects of stress and living in a world of unrelenting tension doesn't mean that the condition is in any way normal, inevitable or untreatable.

On the contrary, the good news is that our conditioned responses can be transformed so completely that life can rapidly become a much more profoundly enjoyable experience. Mastery of the stress response will be one of our most important objectives.

How Females deal with Mid Life Challenges

The Mid Life generation today grew up with choices. This is the generation who grew up with birth control, kitchen technology, contact lenses, plastic surgery, women's lib, one-calorie soda, liposuction, E-mail, and cell phones. This is the generation of women who rewrote the rules:

So if everyone is calling you "Ma'am" and the police are looking younger and younger, welcome to those middle years. Today, the average forty-year-old American woman can expect to live to be at least eighty years old.

Unfortunately, it is during these middle years that many women experience more anxiety and depression than at any other time in their life. Think of the many stresses produced by changing self-concepts, marriage dissatisfaction, redefinition of parenting roles, and the double standard of aging.

How Does Our Aging Experience Compare?

Anti-Inflammatory Diet Your Pathway to Looking and Feeling 10 Years Younger
By Beran Parry

In an article written more than twenty years ago, Susan Sontag described some interesting observations but some of them are changing!

- As they grow older, women often keep their age a secret. Most men do not.
- Since women are often judged on their beauty and youthfulness, their value as partners may decrease as they mature. Since men are often judged on their competence and experience, their value as partners may increase as they mature.
- An older woman is considered less sexually attractive and desirable than a younger woman. An older man, particularly if he is financially or politically successful, does not lose his sexual eligibility. In fact, it often increases as his power increases, and the male/female mortality rates make him a scarce sexual commodity!
- Older men can be expected to take younger lovers; older women are not. But now they are starting to!
- Women are expected to try to maintain facial beauty through cosmetics, moisturizers, and even surgery. Men are expected to have their faces become more rugged, scarred and marked by the passing years.

Men and women do not approach the aging "starting line" neck and neck. Many of the stresses that affect women as they age have begun to form before they are forty.

It is still more often the woman than the man who has postponed or interrupted a career for the convenience of marriage or the necessities of parenting. It is still more often the woman than the man who has assumed a more flexible position when family decisions had to be made in the midst of pros and cons.

Many women who have spent years of their adult lives at home see themselves as "just housewives," though this is an inaccurate and demeaning view. They feel that their job qualifications, social skills, sexual experience and personal style are rusty and dusty! By the time they are approaching forty, they would like to re-enter the world beyond their homes, but are stressed by what they consider their inadequacies.

These generalizations have not changed very much and help to explain why a woman with years of homemaking experience often feels that she has little of value to offer in her later years. The reverse is true: A homemaker typically has experience in accounting, nutrition, paramedical activities, counselling, decorating, catering, social planning, and sometime hiring, firing and even public relations. If she has particularly enjoyed one of these areas, she can begin to focus on her job or career ambitions.

In fact, the older woman is more desirable than her male counterpart, both in the job market and as a mate. Research indicates that women have greater resistance to haemorrhages, many cancers,

Anti-Inflammatory Diet Your Pathway to Looking and Feeling 10 Years Younger
By Beran Parry

heart disease, and brain disease. In fact, according to research cited by the Society for Women's Health Research in Washington, D. C., women also lose less brain tissue and cerebrospinal fluid as they age, making them less vulnerable to age-related changes in mental ability.

(see references at end of chapter)

Some areas of this chapter adapted from the book

The Female Stress Survival Guide (Witikin PHD, G)

It is becoming increasingly clear that chronic inflammation is the root cause of many serious illnesses - including heart disease, many cancers, and Alzheimer's disease. We all know inflammation on the surface of the body as local redness, heat, swelling and pain. It is the cornerstone of the body's healing response, bringing more nourishment and more immune activity to a site of injury or infection. But when inflammation persists or serves no purpose, it damages the body and causes illness. Stress, lack of exercise, genetic predisposition, and exposure to toxins (like secondhand tobacco smoke) can all contribute to such chronic inflammation, but dietary choices play a big role as well. Learning how specific foods influence the inflammatory process is the best strategy for containing it and reducing long-term disease risks.

Andrew Weil MD

Recently a new study was published which looked at the potential mechanisms underlying the specific anti-inflammatory properties of ketosis

For those unfamiliar, a ketogenic diet is one which contains very little – if any – carbohydrate. One classic example of this dietary approach is seen in the Inuit people. The Inuit are indigenous people, who live in the Arctic region.

Alaska, Canada and Greenland all have Inuit populations.

In one of the more famous nutrition stories of recent times, Dr. Vilhjalmur Stefansson ate nothing but meat for one year, after being inspired by living with the Inuit, and seeing their remarkably low rate of disease

This was despite the Inuit's (then) controversial diet of nothing but meat, whether it came from fish or other sources. Stefansson saw no ill effects from a year of an all meat diet, with basically zero carbohydrate. He also consumed no vegetables. It is worth noting, that he also became very ill when he consumed only low fat meat, and nothing else. When he added the fattier meat back in, he immediately felt better.

Anti-Inflammatory Diet Your Pathway to Looking and Feeling 10 Years Younger
By Beran Parry

The many reported benefits of the ketogenic diet include, but are not limited to: less hunger while dieting, improved cognitive function in those who are cognitively impaired, improved LDL cholesterol levels, improved weight loss, and improved levels of HDL cholesterol

This is in addition to the aforementioned anti-inflammatory effects. When we look to the scientific literature, we see that the anti-inflammatory nature of the diet has been studied for many years.

The ketogenic diet has also been established as an adequate anticonvulsant therapy.

This newly published research looks specifically at the ketone metabolite beta-hydroxybutyrate, which seems to inhibit the NLRP3 inflammasome

Since the NLRP3 inflammasome was previously found to have been linked to obesity and inflammation, as well as insulin resistance, inhibiting it would make mechanistic sense. The resultant weight loss and anti-inflammatory effects, commonly seem (at least anecdotally) when adopting a ketogenic diet, would then make sense as well. The NLRP3 inflammasome also drives the inflammatory response in several disorders including autoimmune diseases, type 2 diabetes, Alzheimer's disease, atherosclerosis, and autoinflammatory disorders

Could it all be so simple? Possibly, though there is certainly likely more to be more scientific discoveries, relating to the beneficial effects of this specific dietary approach. Moving away from glucose and instead utilizing ketone bodies as a source of metabolic fuel, results in many profound changes, of which we are only beginning to scratch the surface of, scientifically.

This new discovery will likely be the first of many new findings regarding the ketogenic diet, and its abundance of benefits. If you are looking to adopt a ketogenic approach, simply follow the Paleo Diet, and then lower your carbohydrate intake to below 100g per day.

How low you need to go for optimum quality of life is highly variant, and many people report different results with different amounts of carbohydrates.

In recent years, three excellent clinical studies have been published that utilized what the authors called a Spanish ketogenic Mediterranean diet.

The diet consisted of olive oil, moderate red wine, green vegetables and salads, fish as the primary protein, as well as lean meat, fowl, eggs, shellfish and cheese. (Nuts are also acceptable, although they were not included in these studies.) Notice that absolutely no sugar, flour, whole grains, or legumes were consumed. Fruit was also not included.

Anti-Inflammatory Diet Your Pathway to Looking and Feeling 10 Years Younger
By Beran Parry

What is a Ketogenic diet?

The Ketogenic diet is a low carb, high fat diet with majority of calories provided by fat, minimal carbs and moderate protein. Contrary to the general belief the fat used in Ketogenic diet, essentially from medium chain fatty acids, are not associated with worsening heart and vascular disease. Medium chain fatty acids have a denser energy potential and is easily converted to ATP for cell consumption.

The ketogenic diet is used to manage a variety of conditions such as diabetes, metabolic syndrome, polycystic ovarian syndrome, obesity, hypertension, epilepsy, gastroesophageal reflux disease and irritable bowel syndrome.

Ketogenic diet has been used since 1920s very effectively to control refractory seizures of childhood epilepsy. It fell out of favor after the introduction of Dilantin the anti seizure medication.

What are ketones?

Ketons are produced in the body when the fats are burned. Ketons are primarily used when glucose is not readily available to be used for fuel. By adopting a Ketogenic diet your body adopts to use fat instead of carbohydrates to obtain fuel for cellular daily function.

Ketone bodies can be used for energy source for most of the normal cells. There is growing evidence that ketones have beneficial effects on aging, inflammation, metabolism, cognition and athletic performance.

Our ancestors used Ketogenic type diet during the non-animal based food shortage and it is known that new born that are strictly breast fed go into Ketogenic state and 25% of their energy needs are supplied by ketones. So nature has already adopted itself to adopt to this type of dietary habits.

The main ketones produced that are measurable in the blood or urine are beta hydroxybutyrate (blood), acetoacetate (urine) acetone (breath).

What are the benefits of a low carb, high fat diet namely nutritional ketosis state?

1. Ketones are the preferred fuel source for liver, brain, heart and muscle.
2. Ketosis is an excellent way of loosing body fat
3. By being keto-adapted you generate fuel from dietary fat and body fat but when we consume excess carbohydrate, it is turned into fat and not easily digested to fuel.
4. Natural hunger and appetite control
5. Effortless weight loss and maintenance
6. Mental clarity

Anti-Inflammatory Diet Your Pathway to Looking and Feeling 10 Years Younger
By Beran Parry

7. Better sleep
8. Normalized metabolic function
9. Stabilized blood sugar and increased cellular insulin sensitivity
10. Lower inflammation in the body
11. Blood pressure control
12. Better cholesterol control with increase in good cholesterol (HDL) and decrease in bad cholesterol (LDL) and triglycerides
13. Better fertility
14. Improved immune system
15. Reduction of free radicals and slowing the aging process
16. Improve in cognitive function and memory
17. Decreased anxiety and mood swings
18. Decreased heartburn
19. Felling general well-being and happiness

The application of this diet for 12 weeks led to weight loss and the resolution of metabolic syndrome and non-alcoholic fatty liver disease, demonstrating that a ketogenic diet is highly anti-inflammatory.

Some areas of this chapter adapted from the book

The Female Stress Survival Guide (Witikin PHD, G)

Anti-Inflammatory Diet Your Pathway to Looking and Feeling 10 Years Younger
By Beran Parry

Chapter 6:

10 YEARS YOUNGER

Medical Minimally Invasive Aesthetic Anti-Ageing Procedures

DISCLAIMER: I am not personally advocating any of these treatments, I am simply showing what is available as an alternative to more invasive facial procedures)

As the primary point of contact with others, your face is the first chance available to connect with others and provide a suitable visual to whatever you are communicating about. Whether you're seeking a confidence boost or you simply want to look your best, Anti-aging treatments are minimally-invasive facial rejuvenation options available for both women and men. The results are smooth facial lines, reduced sagging, and corrected skin folds.

Rejuvenate *Your* Appearance

Aesthetic concerns are as unique as a fingerprint, so a one-size-fits-all answer simply doesn't work. Some individuals struggle with fine lines, while others experience loss of elasticity or profound smile lines. No matter your concern, there are multiple solutions to specifically target the problem.

Achieve Results the Same Day

Some facial rejuvenation procedures offer patients visible results as early as the same day and are nearly painless, as injections are given with small needles and the local area is numbed prior to the procedure. Because there is virtually no recovery time and little pain, anti-aging treatments can fit into your schedule without interrupting daily life. Though temporary, the effect lasts for several months without the need for frequent maintenance.

Variety of Prescription Options

Anti-Inflammatory Diet Your Pathway to Looking and Feeling 10 Years Younger
By Beran Parry

With advances in science and technology, multiple anti-aging treatments are available via prescription. In the past, there were few options outside of surgery capable of producing desired results. Men and women were faced with the option of going under the knife or applying ineffective topical treatments. Now, with multiple options available backed by clinical trials, you have access to a prescription designed to specifically address your concerns.

Here are some examples…

Botox is a popular anti-aging non-surgical treatment that involves injecting a diluted version of the botulinum toxin into muscles on the face. The toxin blocks the signal that tells the muscles to contract or cause the skin around the eyes or forehead to wrinkle. Like many other anti-aging non-surgical treatments, Botox is painless and anesthesia is not used. Botox is administered using a fine needle to minimize discomfort. Results typically appear within two to four weeks and last between four to six months. Botox is also used as a treatment for patients suffering from serious medical conditions, such as muscle disorders.

NB – Integrative Medicine does not advocate Botox treatments if there is a history of certain wellbeing issues. Please see an integrative doctor before making any decisions

Chemical Peels: Undergoing a chemical peel is a popular anti-aging non-surgical treatment because it's considered an effective alternative to costly surgery. The procedure involves applying an acid-based solution to small areas of the skin, be it the face, hands, or neck. The solution is typically washed away after two minutes, and to minimize discomfort, a small fan may be directed over the spot where the acid was applied. Depending on the strength of the formula used, it may take several treatments to see any noticeable results. With stronger peels, like phenol peels, the recovery time can be up to three months, because of the severely sunburned look the skin takes on.

CO2 Laser: Laser skin resurfacing is the latest treatment in the fight against aging. This anti-aging non-surgical treatment uses a laser beam that is broken up into many small micro beams to target specific areas, while promoting rapid healing in the untreated areas. In treated areas, the laser promotes the production of collagen. It is an effective treatment for acne scars and for smoothing fine lines and wrinkles. It is also a less invasive alternative to costly facelift surgery. The side effects include redness and swelling; however, these are typically minimal and clear up after a day or two.

Collagen: Collagen is a fibrous protein that is used to treat the signs of aging. Collagen treatments involve one of two procedures. The less invasive collagen facial uses a collagen cream and facial mask to restore naturally occurring proteins in the skin. The other treatment involves injecting collagen directly into the face to fill in wrinkles or to make lips look fuller. This anti-aging non-surgical treatment takes anywhere from a few minutes to an hour, depending on the size of the area being treated. To minimize discomfort, a topical anaesthetic is applied. The results are immediately noticeable and usually last up to six months.

Fraxel: Fraxel is a fractional laser that uses carbon dioxide (CO_2). It is used in the treatment of everything from sun-damaged skin to wrinkles. The procedure involves small microthermal zones, similar to pixels, which encourage the growth of new skin. It involves three to five treatments, spaced out over three to eight weeks. You will typically see results after a week, and they will usually last five to six months. Recovery time following this anti-aging non-surgical treatment is usually one to seven days. Your skin may look red and swollen immediately after your treatment.

GentleWaves: GentleWaves LED photo modulation is the latest method in the fight against aging. Unlike invasive surgical procedures or treatments that use harsh chemicals, GentleWaves uses low-intensity light-emitting diodes (LEDs) to stimulate the skin's production of collagen, resulting in more youthful, rejuvenated skin. Alternately, it also suppresses the enzymes that break down collagen. An LED device is applied to the area to be treated and only takes five minutes. No aftercare is required and the device is compatible with all skin types. It usually takes four to eight treatments to see results with this anti-aging non-surgical treatment, and the procedure is completely painless.

Hyaluronic Acid Fillers: Injectable wrinkle fillers, such as hyaluronic acid fillers, are an affordable option for anyone looking for an alternative to costly and invasive facelift procedures. Hyaluronic acid is a naturally occurring substance that binds to moisture between skin cells. The injections differ from treatments like Botox by filling in wrinkles, as well as volumizing skin for fuller lips, giving cheeks a lift, and plumping sagging skin on the hands. It also has the benefit of reducing the appearance of scars. Hyaluronic acid is injected directly into the area. Like other anti-aging non-surgical treatments, you may experience mild swelling and bruising following the treatment.

Consider checking of you have any contraindications to lidocaine before deciding on these treatments

Intense Pulsed Light (IPL): Intense pulsed light, or IPL, is an anti-aging non-surgical treatment that uses wavelengths of light to correct wrinkles and treat sun-damaged skin. It is also used as a hair removal treatment. The procedure uses intense bursts of light applied to a small area via a handheld device or an articulated lamp. The process triggers a damage-control response in the skin, leading it to shed the old skin and take on a smoother, more youthful appearance. There may be mild pain and discomfort following the procedure. Note that it may take up to 12 treatments before you see any results.

Microdermabrasion: Microdermabrasion has been dubbed "an instant facelift." The procedure, which involves spraying tiny grains to buff away a layer of skin, is far less invasive and much more affordable than facelift surgery. This anti-aging non-surgical treatment triggers an injury response in the

Anti-Inflammatory Diet Your Pathway to Looking and Feeling 10 Years Younger
By Beran Parry

skin, and the body reacts by replacing the skin that was stripped away with smoother, younger-looking skin. The procedure uses a specialized tool that both sprays the grains and cleans up the dead skin. Though you will likely see immediate results, six treatments performed 10 to 14 days apart are recommended for the best outcome. The procedure also reduces the size of pores and the skin's oiliness.

Pulsed-Dye Lasers: Pulsed-dye lasers (PDLs) are an anti-aging non-surgical treatment used for skin conditions such as port-wine stains, scars, spider veins, and more. Before the procedure starts, the dermatologist may do several test patches to determine the best strength for the laser. The laser will then be applied to the area being treated. The process sends short pulses to the area. There may be mild pain, but most of the time; a cooling spray will be applied to minimize any discomfort. PDL treatment only takes a few minutes, and it may require up to three treatments before any results are visible. Bruising is the most common side effect.

Reloxin: Reloxin is an alternative to Botox that achieves the same results. Like Botox, it is derived from botulinum toxin type A. But unlike Botox, the concentration of botulinum isn't as high in Reloxin; therefore, the results are reported to last longer. Like Botox, Reloxin is injected directly into the area being treated using a fine needle to minimize discomfort in the patient. The results typically last anywhere from five to six months. Results also usually appear within one to two days, as opposed to Botox's two to four weeks, making Reloxin a great alternate anti-aging non-surgical treatment.

Retinoids: A lot of people have probably used some form of a retinoid at some point in their life, but without ever knowing it. "Retinoid" is a term used to describe vitamin A derivatives that unclog pores, boost collagen to reduce fine lines, and help smooth the skin. Although as many as 5,000 retinoids have been identified and/or synthesized, the FDA has only approved a few retinoid drugs. The first was approved by the FDA in 1971 for acne use; at the time, dermatologists noticed that patients using retinol had skin that was clearer, softer, and smoother. Retinoids have also been shown to effectively combat wrinkles, speed cell turnover to fade sunspots, and increase the thickness of the dermis (the deep layer of skin where wrinkles form.) Anti-aging non-surgical treatments containing Retinoids are available over the counter, although these may not be as effective as a prescription retinoid.

Sclerotherapy: Varicose veins are enlarged veins near the surface of the skin. While the development of varicose veins and spider veins can occur at any age, they usually surface between the ages of 18 and 35 and peak by age 60. Most common in the legs and ankles, pregnancy is a contributing factor to the formation of varicose veins and spider veins, as is aging. One of the best ways to treat varicose veins and spider veins is with an anti-aging non-surgical treatment called sclerotherapy, a procedure whereby a physician injects a solution (sclerosant) directly into the affected vein. The solution damages and scars the inside lining of the vein, causing it to close. The vein then turns into scar tissue that eventually fades.

Anti-Inflammatory Diet Your Pathway to Looking and Feeling 10 Years Younger
By Beran Parry

Anti-Aging Non-Surgical Treatments Explained

Sculptra: One of the safest, longest-lasting ways to look younger is with an anti-aging non-surgical treatment called Sculptra. Approved by the FDA in 2009 for the correction of shallow to deep smile lines and other facial wrinkles, Sculptra is not a wrinkle filler, but rather, a volumizer. Sculptra works through a series of injections that fill the depressed areas of the face caused by aging (collagen loss). Sculptra is made of a synthetic material known as poly-L-lactic acid, a substance that forms naturally in the body when you exercise. A full Sculptra treatment consists, on average, of three sessions over a few months, and the results can last for more than two years.

Thermage: Thermage is perfect for those who want to address the visible signs of aging in just one treatment. It's an anti-aging non-surgical procedure that's clinically proven to safely treat fine lines and wrinkles on most body parts, including the face, eyes, neck, stomach, arms, hands, thighs, and buttocks. Thermage has even been approved by the FDA for improving cellulite. Thermage uses radio frequency to non-surgically tighten skin and lift problem areas on the body. It heats the deepest layers of skin to help tighten existing collagen and stimulate the natural renewal of collagen. Benefits of Thermage as an anti-aging non-surgical treatment include the smoothing of wrinkly or uneven skin; better definition around the eyes, jaw, and neckline; and the smoothing and toning of unsightly dimples and wrinkles on the face and body.

Thread Lift: For those who don't like the idea of going under the knife, but want the immediate benefits of a surgical neck or facelift, there's the minimally invasive thread lift, also known as a suture lift or stitch lift. As the name implies, the procedure uses "threads" made out of specialized suture material to lift the skin of the eyebrows, mid-face, cheeks, and neck. Unlike facelifts, thread lifts are anti-aging non-surgical treatments; thread lifts are performed using a local anesthetic. Bandages are not required after a thread lift, and recovery time is just two to three days.

Titan: Titan skin rejuvenation is an infrared laser treatment that uses light energy to stimulate new collagen growth deep beneath the skin's surface. Titan has been shown to tighten skin on your face, arms, abdomen, and legs. A Titan procedure has also been shown to resurface the skin, tighten pores, remove age spots, and smooth away fine lines. While some patients report seeing results in as few as one or two procedures, the full benefits of the Titan procedure are not usually observed for at least three to six months. The Titan procedure is considered an ideal alternative to those who want to enhance their youthful appearance without invasive surgery, prolonged recovery time, or injections.

This chapter is adapted from an article on agein.com website (Bawa, S)

Anti-Inflammatory Diet Your Pathway to Looking and Feeling 10 Years Younger
By Beran Parry

Anti-Inflammatory Diet Your Pathway to Looking and Feeling 10 Years Younger
By Beran Parry

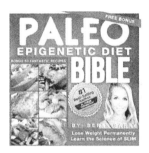

Chapter 7:

Epigenetics + Long Term Eating Behaviours = Your Present Weight Level

How the eating habits we acquired in the past profoundly affect our food choices today. How Genetics are no longer the prime influence on our health and wellbeing Epigenetics provides us with the insights, analysis, tools and strategies for permanent healthy weight loss.

We really believe that knowledge is power and we want you to understand as much about this important subject as possible. Being armed with the best information will strengthen your understanding of how to master your weight issues, take away all that ridiculous and unnecessary guilt about being overweight and prepare you for a newer, happier, skinnier you.

Perhaps you haven't heard all the excitement in medical and scientific circles about the latest revelations in the field of Epigenetics. Epi-what? OK. Before we go any further, you're probably wondering what on earth Epigenetics really means. Is it contagious? Can we get it at the grocery store? Does it come in my size? So let's start by answering an important question: "What exactly is Epigenetics?"

The formal description of Epigenetics from the text books refers to the study of changes in organisms caused by modification of gene expression rather than by an alteration of the genetic code itself. That might not tell us very much but it really is an important statement! It's no longer simply a case of identifying which particular genes you have.

Anti-Inflammatory Diet Your Pathway to Looking and Feeling 10 Years Younger
By Beran Parry

We now know that it's the way your genes are influenced and made to work that makes the difference. Gene expression accounts for so many of our characteristics. And changes in gene expression have been related to a very wide range of environmental influences and that includes – are you ready for this? – What we eat!

Yes, that's absolutely right. The kind of food we consume every single day, the quality of the food we eat, the eating choices we make all contribute far more to our total health and wellbeing than was ever appreciated before. It's not a question of being pre-programmed by our DNA. We've been bombarded by articles and news items for decades telling us every day that everything in our lives is caused by our genes.

But what if it isn't just the genetic luck of the draw? What if our health is connected far more to how we live, to what we eat and a whole range of external factors that we can influence? What if we're not programmed to be fat? What if it's about the choices we make? It's becoming increasingly clear that the choices we make really are incredibly important to our health and wellbeing. This means we really can influence our health right now right down to the cellular level and that obviously includes our weight as well. This is the breakthrough in our understanding that is revolutionising our entire approach to health and weight control. Our genes do not determine our weight. The answer is not in your genetic code. It's on the end of your fork!

So when we consult the latest reference works in this exciting new area of scientific research, we find that Epigenetics demonstrates the importance of influences which are firmly outside the traditional genetic system. This is the conclusion of Lyle Armstrong, whose research programme is widely respected at the Institute of Genetic Medicine at Newcastle University in the United Kingdom.

Modern biology is rewriting our understanding of genetics, disease and inherited characteristics. This is the view of Nessa Carey in her fascinating book "The Epigenetics Revolution".

This means that our understanding is also undergoing a revolution. The popular media still love to produce stories every day telling us that so many health problems are simply the result of your unlucky genes. But that's practically medieval in terms of medical science. We now know that we really can take the necessary steps to regain control of our general health, our health concerns and our weight. This must be one of the most important medical discoveries of the age.

Let's also bear in mind that science is not a fixed commodity.

In an age of extraordinary technological advances, our knowledge and understanding of how the human body functions are being tested and challenged every single day. That's why research is so important. And research changes the way we understand everything. This revolutionary development in our understanding of how the body really works is laying the foundation for all future medical analysis

Anti-Inflammatory Diet Your Pathway to Looking and Feeling 10 Years Younger
By Beran Parry

and treatment. The epigenetics principle represents one of the most important changes in how we are going to manage health issues in the future, from disease prevention to maintaining long term health.

The exciting thing is that we don't have to wait for the future to take full advantage of these discoveries. We are going to use it to get healthier and skinnier right now! We are going to show you the smart way to take control of your weight, and it's the way your body will love the most. We're going to help you to get into the best shape of your life. And we're going to show you how to stay that way.

What does this mean for you right now? Well, let's see if we can re-cap the essentials of the Epigenetics revolution.

To start, we know that our genes definitely gave us a set of fixed characteristics. Eye colour, height and bone structure are examples of pre-determined characteristic donated by the genes you inherited from your parents.

But many areas of your life and wellbeing can be determined by the choices you make.

Weight control is a perfect example of this discovery. We now know that life span and the risk of contracting many diseases can be influenced by how we live our lives. The way we eat, the chemicals we absorb, the stress levels we endure all contribute to our health profiles and, most importantly, can change the way our DNA behaves. These minor alterations in gene behaviour can work in our favour or they can most certainly work against us. They can even be passed onto future generations.

So we have a direct responsibility for our own health and wellbeing and also for the welfare of future children and grandchildren. If you're interested in the technical background to this amazing phenomenon, the critical factor is a chemical code known as the epigenome.

This chemical coating surrounds your DNA and can switch certain genes off and on. So Epigenetics is primarily concerned with the study of this chemical layer and how it influences the way our genes function. Studies demonstrate that our genes only suggest what might happen in terms of our future health issues; our behaviour is much more important in determining the outcomes.

"There's nothing you can do about your DNA, but you can influence the way it functions by changing your lifestyle," says Ajay Goel, Ph.D., Director of Epigenetics and Cancer Prevention at Baylor Research Institute.

As a great example of how important this discovery has been for future health issues, even if you have a family history of certain kinds of cancer, eating particular foods can instruct the epigenome to switch off the cancer-prone genes.

Anti-Inflammatory Diet Your Pathway to Looking and Feeling 10 Years Younger
By Beran Parry

You might want to read that sentence again.

The message is just too important to miss. This is the moment when the tide of obesity turns. This is when we recognise that we need to change our metabolic function as well as our food intake. This is when we finally take control of our weight issues. Now is the time to accept responsibility for our health and wellbeing and take the necessary steps to put things right. And keep them right.

If you're still keeping track of the technical data behind these revolutionary studies, you might like to know a little more about another influence on gene behaviour - methylation. This is a really interesting area of research but you might not want to make it your specialist subject when you go to parties! It's an incredibly important topic but most people, especially the ones who prefer to believe that they're just the unfortunate victims of their ill-fated DNA, probably don't want to have their illusions shattered. But you will know. And knowledge, my friend, especially this kind of knowledge is power.

Diet is a much easier subject to study than stress or other behaviours. It's been much easier to explore the effects of diet on epigenetics than the effects of the wider environment. So we know a great deal about the way food impacts on our genes.

Intelligent nutrition and appropriate exercise promote efficient fat-burning, healthy muscle building, longevity and wellness. Using your body's natural ability to respond to good nutrition, we can turn away forever from the nightmare of gaining and storing fat and losing muscle mass. We can reduce the risk of disease and illness. A brighter future beckons. This is the promise of Epigenetics.

As we mentioned before, our physical characteristics are largely based on our parents' DNA. Protecting your DNA from malfunction is not a luxury option any more. It's an essential task for all of us to undertake to ensure better health, quality of life and sustainable wellbeing.

Dr Trygve Tollefsbol wrote in the 2010 edition of Clinical Epigenetics that adding methyl-modifying compounds to the diet can help reduce the incidence and severity of disease. So we know from all the evidence that is being produced on a daily basis that you can reprogram your genes to favour weight loss, improve overall health and boost longevity by following three very simple procedures. You might want to print out these ideas and put them on your fridge door right now!

Anti-Inflammatory Diet Your Pathway to Looking and Feeling 10 Years Younger
By Beran Parry

The 10 YEARS YOUNGER Three Golden Food Rules!

1. Weight loss is all about insulin

Moderate your insulin production levels by eliminating sugar and grains (yes, even whole grains) and you will lose the excess body fat without dieting - plus you will improve your energy levels, reduce inflammation throughout the body and eliminate disease risk. Maybe this should be printed in a very large font size in the brightest colour your printer can produce!

2. Eating lean protein but plenty good quality fat

Vegetable and some correctly sourced animal protein with high good fat content are not only healthy but are the keys to effortless weight loss, a healthy immune system and boundless energy.

3. Eat Clean

When we examine the role that food plays in avoiding or encouraging weight gain, you might be shocked to discover that one of the biggest influences is concealed in the way that our food is processed. Hold onto your hat, my friend. This can get scary! The most significant components of food that play the largest role in weight gain and obesity are food additives, chemicals, and food processing techniques.

These principles are sacred and mark the beginning of your transformation. They are so important that they need to be practised and respected every single day. They are the foundation for much of the change we are creating. You could finish the book first but the only time you have to begin the revolution is right now. So let's make the commitment right this instant to use these golden principles and kick start the new life we've been waiting for. And I mean right now!

Epigenetic research has been at the forefront of these discoveries and that's why the methods in this book respect the need to resolve all of the issues surrounding intelligent, effective, permanent weight control.

Some Excellent eating Programs that positively contribute to Correct Epigenetic eating

We live in a world of fascinating research and fast-paced developments, instant communication, masses of information and an explosion in obesity rates. Somewhere along the line in our very recent history something has gone dramatically wrong. Part of the response to this weighty problem has been an explosion in the number of diet books and diet plans and weight loss organisations. But the problem is still as large as it ever was. And so many people find that even when they've managed to lose some

Anti-Inflammatory Diet Your Pathway to Looking and Feeling 10 Years Younger
By Beran Parry

weight, it goes back on in a flash. We did not evolve to be chronically overweight. Nature equipped us with incredibly efficient bodies. Clearly we need a better approach to this problem. We need an approach that works. We need a method that will give us sustainable results. So let's take a look at some of the more recent innovations in weight control technology.

The Paleo Diet

The theory is that many of our current health problems are a result of our modern eating habits. There's been a great deal of publicity surrounding the growing view that we simply haven't evolved to the point where we can safely consume a grain-rich diet. Our distant ancestors in the Old Stone Age or Paleolithic Era consumed a very different diet compared to modern humans because they simply didn't have access to agriculture. That's because agriculture didn't exist. It hadn't been invented. The typical caveman's food was natural, unprocessed, varied, seasonal and a result of labour-intensive, hunter-gathering activities.

The Paleo approach to nutrition recognises that we've only been consuming grains for the last ten thousand years or so. That's a long wait at the bus stop but it really is not long enough in evolutionary terms for humans to have adapted to this radical shift in eating behaviour. The modern diet is heavily reliant on grains and dairy products and suffers from a toxic surfeit of sugar. Grains were the mechanism that allowed for a more predictable food supply and those ancient crop surpluses provided the essential catalyst from which the seeds of civilisation sprang. The problem, as you now know only too well, is that grains damage the gut, weaken the immune system and degrade our health.

The Paleo alternative recognises how our digestive system works and focuses on providing the best quality fuel for our bodies. That includes fresh fruits, vegetables, lean meat, eggs and nuts. No grains. No processed sugars. No milk products. Paleo has scored very highly as a weight control mechanism because this kind of diet suits our evolutionary history so well. When we adapt our eating habits to this more natural way of getting our daily calories, our metabolisms shift from carb-burning to fat-burning. No surprise then that the Paleo diet has become a favourite tool for encouraging serious weight loss and for enhancing better levels of health.

The focus is on natural, unprocessed food and it is this emphasis on eating as naturally as possible that is the key to the method's success. As you might expect in a new way of approaching our food needs, the Paleo diet has spawned a number of variations and alternatives. Some enthuslasts avoid all forms of dairy produce whilst others are convinced that some specific dairy products are essential. The wisdom of avoiding grains though is widely accepted by most Paleo devotees.

Anti-Inflammatory Diet Your Pathway to Looking and Feeling 10 Years Younger
By Beran Parry

The Growing Younger Take on the Paleo Diet

You might recognise some aspects of the Paleo Diet in our advice in this book. It certainly has some interesting and relevant merits in terms of getting the body into great shape and the emphasis on pure protein and natural, unprocessed vegetables is a key to restoring the intestinal flora to its healthiest and most effective condition.

The Vegan Option

In a world of unhealthy and even toxic food choices, we shouldn't be surprised that the Vegan diet is associated with lots of positive health benefits. Vegans typically experience lower cholesterol levels, lower blood pressure and less body fat than their meat-eating counterparts. And this might be an important clue about the Vegan success story. If we've been consuming garbage consistently for years and our bodies are suffering from toxic overload, the Vegan diet is a great way to cleanse, heal and restore the digestive system to its natural condition and give our bodies a welcome break from the daily diet of tasty toxins.

But is it enough to sustain long-term, normal health?

Vegans don't eat meat or dairy products. The typical consumer in the developed world eats vast amounts of processed food, especially meat and dairy. Is it simply a question of removing all meat and dairy products from our daily diet or is it more effective to reduce our total intake and only eat lean, unprocessed meat with limited quantities of specific dairy products?

The answer might be found in our evolutionary history. Vegans miss out on a wide range of nutrients because humans evolved to eat a broad range of foodstuffs. As a species, we certainly thrive on fresh fruit and vegetables but we also benefit from the occasional meal of animal protein. If we miss out on the essential fats in our diet, our bodies can't metabolise protein effectively.

Vegans might be missing out on several key nutrients and perhaps the simplest answer to these deficiencies can be found in taking lots of supplements. Iron deficiency, lack of Vitamin D, insufficient iodine, low Vitamin B levels, low Vitamin A and low zinc levels are all associated with the Vegan diet. But let's be clear - many Vegans lead a very healthy, energy-filled life and have adapted perfectly to this form of diet.

It's also true that many people experience long-term issues with this diet due to the limited range of their food choices. As always, the answer will depend on the individual and on whether the diet is sustainable over the long term. And let's also bear in mind that many Vegans commit to their diet choice on moral grounds and refuse to eat anything that involves the exploitation of animals in any form. Their lifestyle is not just a diet. It's a philosophy and a way of life and we need to respect the motivation, passion and commitment that fuels their decision to live as a Vegan, even when that choice results in possible negative consequences for their health.

The Growing Younger Take on the Vegan system

You might have recognised some aspects of the Vegan Diet in our advice in this manual. It certainly has some interesting and relevant merits in terms of getting the body into great shape. The emphasis on natural, unprocessed vegetables is a key to restoring the intestinal flora to its healthiest and most effective condition. Read more about this in our Skinny Delicious Eating Selection Pyramid later on.

Intermittent Fasting

There is a long-established tradition in many cultures that we can live longer and certainly experience better health by fasting on a regular basis. Fasting however takes many forms. At one extreme, it can involve total abstention from food for an extended period of time and this technique has been used to treat a range of severe illnesses including many forms of cancer.

Conducted under strict medical supervision, this form of extreme fasting with close monitoring in a controlled, clinical environment has produced extraordinary results in severely ill patients. There are several theories explaining why the technique is so effective but it is sufficient to know that certain elements of the medical fraternity have been using the method successfully for several decades.

It seems that the body possesses latent powers of healing and regeneration that are triggered during this form of controlled starvation. But it should only ever be attempted under the advice and supervision of experienced, medical professionals.

The Growing Younger Take on Intermittent Fasting

On a lighter scale, fasting can involve abstaining from solid food for twelve to twenty-four hours whilst drinking lots of liquids, soups and juices.

Obviously energy levels can suffer during fasting and some people experience initial unpleasant side effects as the body flushes out the old toxins and restores a more natural balance to the digestive system. The results are usually extremely worthwhile and most people feel a surge of new energy as well as visible changes in their skin and overall condition.

Intermittent fasting is a safe and effective method for re-setting the body's metabolic system and for re-balancing those critical insulin levels. All from simple fasting. The best approach is to try it for one meal three or four times a week

Anti-Inflammatory Diet Your Pathway to Looking and Feeling 10 Years Younger
By Beran Parry

Our Skinny Delicious Detox Program introduces a gentle, easy but effective way to employ Intermittent Fasting to help you lose weight effectively and safely!

The fact is that we are surrounded by toxins at every level and a simple regime of regular fasting is one of the best ways to flush the garbage out of your system. It's got to be one your strongest methods for experiencing total wellbeing and supercharging your weight loss program at the same time!.

In our plan you will learn exactly how to apply these excellent eating regimes to benefit you according to your individual epigenetic needs. Here are some general ideas which we incorporate into your Growing Younger Planning.

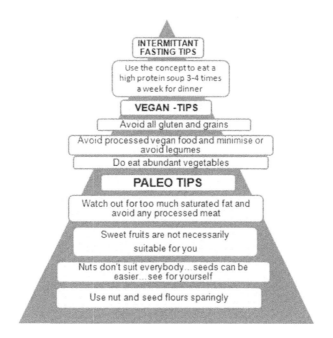

Anti-Inflammatory Diet Your Pathway to Looking and Feeling 10 Years Younger
By Beran Parry

Summary - Epigenetics

Your genetic profile is not the full story

Your genes can be switched on and off

The food you eat is the key to influencing your genetic responses

Methylation and diet change the rules of the genetic game

Managing insulin levels by eliminating all grains

Eat Lean, Clean and Good fats

Take practical steps to address food addiction

Anti-Inflammatory Diet Your Pathway to Looking and Feeling 10 Years Younger
By Beran Parry

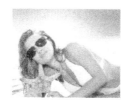

Chapter 8:

Introduction to The 10 YEARS YOUNGER Skin Beauty in Midlife

There is no such thing as an ugly woman.

You deserve to love yourself and accept who you are!

All women are beautiful. You are beautiful, you are fabulous, we all are beautiful but the question is how do I reflect this beauty on my face, hair, body and soul? The answer is easy and doesn't need a lot of effort and money. All you need is few minutes of your time each day. Yes, just a few minutes each day so let's get started right now!

The skin types vary from person to person. Some have dry skin; some have oily skin while others have normal skin. My goal here is to help you to get your skin looking fabulous and rejuvenated using natural products from your kitchen! Yes, everyday household or kitchen items are the thing you can use to create glowing and healthy skin.

Not only can you treat your skin, no matter what type it may be, you can treat your hair with food items as well. No matter what products you find out there you will find a home treatment that is just as effective or even more so. For instance, women have been using Knox gelatin for many, many years to strengthen their nails. When they say beauty comes from the inside it is not just about the soul of a woman. The foods you eat affect the health of your body including your nails, skin and hair.

When it comes to choosing products for your face, skin, nails and hair you probably have found there are unlimited sources of products all claiming to be better than the next. Some are extremely expensive and tough to fit into the average budget today and others that may be cheap really do not do the job as you might expect. What do you do?

Anti-Inflammatory Diet Your Pathway to Looking and Feeling 10 Years Younger
By Beran Parry

We all realize that taking good care of our health is a very important task but did you know that eating correctly and exercising is also a way to bring out your natural beauty? What I am about to share with you is not one of the latest fads that celebrities use or some ridiculously expensive new tonic that celebrities say they use.

Foods that Improve your Appearance from the Inside Out

Foods that will improve your general health will also improve your healthy appearance. A healthy glow is always a very attractive quality. Of course there are the obvious choices like eating plenty of green leafy vegetables. These are considered complex carbohydrates or 'slow' carbs which are excellent for your body. They take a long time to be processed in your system and contain vitamins and iron that is essential for healthy skin, nails and hair. Using balance in your diet with a combination of both vegetable carbohydrates, proteins, and good fats will not only bring health to your body but will enhance your outer beauty.

You want to eat foods every day that contain vitamins, minerals, antioxidants and iron to keep your body healthy and to keep it functioning correctly. Digestive problems can cause your body to build up toxins in the system that in an effort to leave the body can cause blemishes.

Consuming the following foods will not only help your overall health but will specifically help your outer appearance.

---- Supple Skin ----

Apple cider vinegar will really do wonderful things for your system. Some say it helps your body process sugar and fat which helps in weight control. For your skin it is wonderful because it helps to give it that supple quality. The experts say that it also helps in the shedding of dead skin. You can mix a teaspoon to a tablespoon in your juice or drink it straight if you can tolerate the taste. Organic apple cider vinegar is the optimum choice.

---- Prevent Premature Aging ----

Carrots: Vegetables like the green leafy ones we mentioned and other vegetables like carrots are important. The carotene in carrots is said to help to prevent premature aging. Known for their ability to improve eyesight they are also great for regulating the sugars in your body, detoxifying your liver which will help to prevent blemishes. Carrots are also a good source for the vitamins your body needs for healthy skin and hair. *Carrots contain a large amount of vitamin A plus other nutrients that are wonderful nourishing agents for the skin and do prevent dry skin. The list of benefits from eating carrots is impressive.*

Anti-Inflammatory Diet Your Pathway to Looking and Feeling 10 Years Younger
By Beran Parry

Apples: Have you heard the expression, "an apple a day keeps the doctor away"? For skin that is youthful in appearance, you cannot beat the benefits of eating apples, especially Red Delicious and Granny Smith. Not only will eating apples help with the elasticity of your skin but can help to protect damage to your skin from UV rays. Apples contain procyanidin B-2 which is known to promote hair growth and help in the prevention of cell damage.

---- **Urinary Tract Health** ----

Cranberries: Consuming cranberry juice or eating cranberries will help with your urinary tract health.

---- **Prevent Wrinkles** ----

Garlic is something you can eat to help stop your skin from wrinkling because it restores tissues.

Another great food for preventing wrinkles from forming is ***Sweet Potatoes***. They are loaded with vitamin A which does wonders for your skin in general. Your skin will be smoother and clearer. Sweet potatoes do not have the starch that the white potato has so it is a much healthier choice all around.

Foods that have natural bacteria like ***Hard Cheeses*** can prevent cavities and help stop bacteria growth in the mouth.

Other foods containing natural bacteria like ***Yogurt*** can help with your digestive health. Sugar can actually add to the problems of a yeast infection. The yogurt also is great for fighting tooth decay and helps to keep your teeth whiter.

Vitamins A, C and potassium (great for skin and hair): Consuming citrus type fruits will help the body form collagen which holds the skin cells together. *Be sure to include citrus fruit in your daily diet for its other health benefits like lots of vitamin C.*

Tomatoes which are a fruit rather than a vegetable like most think are also great for the skin and contain quantities of vitamins A, C and potassium.

Avocados are also a good source of potassium. They contain natural oils and vitamins that help both your skin and your hair.

<u>**Hair care:**</u> Bananas help to protect the elasticity of the hair which prevents the ends from splitting and it makes the hair soft and strong preventing breakage. Bananas keep the hair shiny and help it grow. They control dandruff and are great for repairing damaged hair while adding volume to the hair.

Anti-Inflammatory Diet Your Pathway to Looking and Feeling 10 Years Younger
By Beran Parry

Skin care: Actually just rubbing the peel of the banana on the skin, especially where there are any irritations like acne or insect bites can be very beneficial. Using the pulp of the banana directly on the face by mashing it up and spreading it on will help to make the skin soft and supple as well.

Chapter 9:

Getting Organised!

Lets start Re-Organising Your Permanent Weight Reduction and Growing Younger Disgracefully Pathway to Permanent Weightloss!

Time to re-programme your food choices and eating behaviour

We are going to learn how to:

Exorcise the past and be free of old habits

Why we prioritise our activities in the wrong order

I've heard it so often, it's almost become the mantra of the unwilling, the permanent excuse for letting things slide. "There just isn't enough time to eat healthily and plan special meals, let alone shop or cook them or take them with me when I'm out of the house."

Sound familiar? Here are more excuses:

I feel so awful when I've eaten badly.

I feel such a failure.

My life is a mess.

Why is it such a struggle to lose weight?"

The result is a fairly miserable outlook and a lack of confidence, an unwillingness to recognise what is possible. The mind-set of the victim. But we're here to address these issues. We want you to feel the confidence that comes from daily, planned success. And getting organised takes all the pain and doubt from the process.

The irony is that the people who claim there's no time to incorporate these important changes in their lives have often been completely successful in other areas of their lives. Their success shows up in an infinite number of ways: they were incredibly accomplished managers or employees, highly creative artistic individuals, massively good parents or even someone who was good at something else. Every

Anti-Inflammatory Diet Your Pathway to Looking and Feeling 10 Years Younger
By Beran Parry

time you make a decision to do something, you're engaging your creative power. All we have to do is harness that potential.

Unhappiness can undoubtedly play its part in the way we treat our bodies. If you have doubts about your self-worth - I know, welcome to the human condition! - It often shows up in unhealthy eating habits and poor choices. It's a huge area and so important that it will be the subject of a future book.

That's why I'd like to encourage you to do something incredibly powerful right now. I want you to look in the mirror for a few moments. And smile. That's right. Smile. Look at yourself and smile. Your conscious mind might feel that the act is a little silly but your subconscious - and your body - will begin to get the message that you're giving them your personal stamp of approval. Have you ever noticed how a small child lights up when you really smile at them? Your body needs exactly that same recognition, that same high wattage smile of approval. Do it every time you step into the bathroom. Look into the mirror and smile. The results will amaze you.

We want your body and your subconscious to work with you. Give them that dazzling smile and you will find your body begins to co-operate in the most extraordinary ways. Try it. It's a very powerful technique for removing behavioural obstacles and we want to make this entire process as easy and comfortable as possible.

This entire book is designed to help you take control of your health, your weight and ultimately your happiness. Being kind to yourself, respecting the miracle of your body, learning to enjoy living in such an extraordinary structure, optimising its potential and being at peace with yourself. These are powerful keys to a very fulfilling way of experiencing the gift of life.

So the underlying theme to these methods is to be kind to yourself. To do things that benefit rather than harm your health. To respect your body's needs and live life to the full.

An abiding love and acceptance of yourself, despite all the imperfections, really helps you to overcome any harmful habits and behaviours and puts an end to the self-criticism and self-loathing that lowers self esteem and sabotages our efforts. It really is extraordinary how quickly we can change our lives simply by learning to accept ourselves and focus not on what might be amiss but on how we truly want to be.

1. Identify your behaviours and habits.

Take a moment. Listen to that inner voice, the way you speak to yourself; check the way you feed yourself; think about your hygiene and sleeping habits.

Anti-Inflammatory Diet Your Pathway to Looking and Feeling 10 Years Younger
By Beran Parry

Which of these areas makes you feel uncomfortable in any way?

Allowing yourself to eat unhealthy food because there just wasn't the time or opportunity to make the effort

Believing that the needs of others are more important than taking care of your body and your weight

Eating food that isn't good for you at any time

Eating late at night or just eating too much

Eating while standing up, out of the package, staring at a computer screen or watching TV

If you catch yourself in the cycle of doing something that you really know you shouldn't, it's an important indicator that there are unresolved issues at work in the subconscious that continue to influence your behaviour.

2. Think about the real consequences of your behaviour.

You might discover that these behaviours and habits are very effective at preventing you from having the things you really want, particularly in terms of having a fit and healthy body that you can really appreciate.

In every moment we are thinking, feeling and doing things that either bring us closer to the person we want to be and the life we want to have or our behaviours take us away from those precious possibilities.

Behaviours ultimately reflect how we really feel about ourselves. Learn to accept yourself right now and the process of transformation will flow so much more smoothly. Learn to smile at yourself and your deeper resources will turn their power towards your new, healthier goals and desires.

3. Learn to understand where your habits came from.

So much of our behaviour was laid down during our early childhoods that we completely forget how we came to be the way we are. Much of our conditioning is no more than a series of programmed reflexes that were given to us at a very impressionable age and those behaviours have survived in our attitudes, thoughts, feelings and beliefs ever since.

Anti-Inflammatory Diet Your Pathway to Looking and Feeling 10 Years Younger
By Beran Parry

Whether they are entirely appropriate can only be measured in terms of whether you're really experiencing all the health, self expression and happiness that is available to you. Most people are not. Sad. But true. Take a look around you. Not too many happy smiling faces, are there? I rest my case. If you're feeling unhappy, comfort is something that is obviously missing and food is one of the easiest sources of a temporary quick fix.

Yes. We're talking chocolate here! So many people reach for the chocolate for an instant rush of pleasure, a way to escape the reality of a stressed and unfulfilled life. Pure comfort food. And I like chocolate too. The intention always seems positive. You give yourself a measure of much needed comfort and an ounce of joy. Unfortunately, it isn't the healthiest way to give yourself those things and it comes with the undesired effects of insulin spikes, sugar crashes and inevitable weight gain followed by a bout of guilt and quiet despair! There has to be a better way. (There is a better way to eat chocolate too...I promise!)

As adults, we're expected to understand the consequences of engaging in a particular thought or behaviour but we often do it anyway. The motivation is always moving away from pain or increasing pleasure. And so many of these actions are a product of that early (and now unconscious) conditioning. It's as if the adult has to be driven so often by a rebellious four year old! No wonder much of our behaviour doesn't make sense. No wonder we don't always behave like truly responsible grown ups.

Comfort food can be very satisfying. We know that many unhealthy behaviours feel good in the short-term (the sugar rush, the comfort, the satisfaction) but we have to recognise that they have long-term detrimental effects. There can also be that familiar hint of the rebel, the thrill of ignoring good advice and breaking the rules. What is it about ourselves that prompts us to do really things to our bodies?

Awareness is very helpful in these circumstances. Spotting the moment when you get a kick from doing the wrong thing helps you to question what's really happening. The adult gets a chance to intervene and make a better choice. That moment when you pause for an instant and wonder why you're doing something, even wondering who is really making the decision. Consciously and deliberately making a wiser, healthier choice. Feeling really good because you've done the right thing. A positive feedback loop that reinforces good behaviour, good choices, adult decisions.

4. Create "house meal planning and eating rules."

Parents make rules because they understand that their children might not have the right perspective for good judgement. Parents can see the consequences that are usually beyond the child's range of experience.

Anti-Inflammatory Diet Your Pathway to Looking and Feeling 10 Years Younger
By Beran Parry

If you have a particularly hard habit to break and you know it's not good for your well-being, consider making it a "house rule" never to have that habit in the home. When something is non-negotiable it removes the inner dialogue where we bargain with ourselves and the simple rule reinforces the right decisions.

5. Develop your powers of awareness.

Be kind to yourself. Most people don't respond well to punishment. Treat yourself gently and with consideration. You've embarked on an important journey and that requires courage and a large measure of recognition.

Be infinitely patient with yourself, as you would be with a child. If you slip up once, instead of throwing everything out the window, learn to accept the failure and resolve to do better.

Understand why you did what you did. What did you need in that moment? Use your new set of rules to support your new behaviour. The rules are your friends. They are there to help you.

What are your new "house eating rules"? How can you maintain your new habits in a way that is supportive, effective and nurturing?

Here are some examples:

1. I always make sure that I have the healthy foods I love at home by doing the shopping myself or by having someone do the shopping for me
2. I always make sure that I have a healthy snack available to me in my refrigerator at all times
3. I always call restaurants ahead of time to order my personal food requirements so that I won't feel uncomfortable when I get there
4. I always take healthy snacks with me to avoid temptation
5. I never allow myself to get too hungry and then I won't have an excuse to eat unhealthy food

These tried and tested methods allow you to exercise control over your feelings and your environment, removing many of the challenging decisions about food choices by making one powerful, healthy choice for all future situations. As you become more aware of how you feel, catching yourself thinking, feeling and about to do things that are no longer in line with your new commitment to total health, you can let go of the old behaviour and make really great choices that will support your vision of a newer, healthier, happier, skinnier you!

Anti-Inflammatory Diet Your Pathway to Looking and Feeling 10 Years Younger
By Beran Parry

Summary - Getting organised

Identify your behaviours and eating choices

Learn to understand the real consequences of your behaviours

Accept your body and start to treat yourself with kindness and understanding

Identify where your habits and behaviours came from

Set up house rules and meal planning schedules

Switch on your awareness

Anti-Inflammatory Diet Your Pathway to Looking and Feeling 10 Years Younger
By Beran Parry

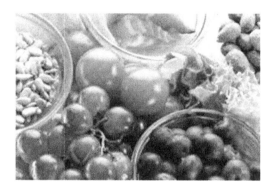

Chapter 10:

GUT BIOLOGY

Your gut biology and the secrets of effective, sustained weight loss

Let's get right down to the guts of the matter! Whilst countless diet books have focused on fads and fleeting feeding fashions, we've had to wait until now to discover that the key to successful weight control is hidden in our intestinal flora. Encouraging the right balance of microbes in our gut and enhancing natural digestion are two of the most important and positive contributions we can make towards generating great health and real weight control.

There is an ancient tradition in many cultures that our intelligence is not simply located in the brain. You might find it surprising that recent research is taking a fresh look at this unusual question and producing some unexpected answers.

Dr Natasha Campbell Macbride, an authority in this fascinating area, states "The importance of your gut flora, and its influence on your health cannot be overstated. It is truly profound. Your gut literally serves as your second brain and even produces more of the neurotransmitter serotonin - known to have a beneficial influence on your mood - than your brain does".

Anti-Inflammatory Diet Your Pathway to Looking and Feeling 10 Years Younger
By Beran Parry

It gets better.

Your gut is also home to countless bacteria, both good and bad. These bacteria outnumber the cells in your body by at least ten to one. We refer to the world of your intestinal flora as the microbiome.

Your microbiome is closely inter-connected with both of your brain systems. Yes. We're proceeding on the basis that we have two locations for the body's operating systems. In addition to the brain in your head, embedded in the wall of your gut is the enteric nervous system (ENS), which works both independently of and in conjunction with the brain in your head.

According to New Scientist: "The ENS is part of the autonomic nervous system, the network of peripheral nerves that control visceral functions. It is also the original nervous system, emerging in the first vertebrates over 500 million years ago and becoming more complex as vertebrates evolved, possibly even giving rise to the brain itself."

Our ancient enteric nervous system is thought to be largely responsible for your "gut instincts," responding to environmental threats and sending information to your brain that directly affects your well-being. I'm sure you've experienced various sensations in your gut that accompany strong emotions such as fear, excitement and stress. Feeling "butterflies" in your stomach is actually the result of blood being diverted away from your gut to your muscles, as part of the fight or flight response.

These reactions in your gut happen outside of your conscious awareness because they are part of your autonomic nervous system, just like the beating of your heart. Your ENS contains around 500 million neurons. Why so many? Because eating is potentially fraught with danger: "Like the skin, the gut must stop potentially dangerous invaders, such as bacteria and viruses, from getting inside the body". This sounds like a perfectly helpful defence mechanism to foster our survival. And what better place to locate a defensive system to protect the body than in the very spot where food can cause the most damage: the gut.

Evolution really has been generous in equipping us with so many ways to keep us safe. If a pathogen should cross the gut lining, immune cells in the gut wall secrete inflammatory substances, including histamine, which are detected by neurons in the ENS. The gut brain then either triggers diarrhoea or alerts the brain in the head, which may decide to initiate vomiting, or both. In other words, the reactions in the gut will send instructions to purge the system as rapidly as possible.

We now know that this communication link between your "two brains" runs in both directions and is the main pathway for the way that foods affect your mood. For example, fatty foods make you feel good because fatty acids are detected by cell receptors in the lining of your gut, which then send warm and fuzzy nerve signals to your brain. Knowing this, you can begin to understand how not only your physical health but also your mental health is deeply influenced by the state of your gut and the

Anti-Inflammatory Diet Your Pathway to Looking and Feeling 10 Years Younger
By Beran Parry

microbial zoo that lives there. Your intestinal microbes affect your overall brain function, so this means that your eating behaviour is also affected by the health of your gut!

When it comes to Inflammation, Your Microbiome Rules

Scientists have found a specific pattern of intestinal microbes that can measurably increase your risk for Type 2 diabetes. This pattern can serve as a biomarker for diabetes probability. Similarly, researchers have also found marked differences in bacterial strains between overweight and non-overweight people. A strain of beneficial bacteria called Lactobacillus rhamnosus has been identified as being helpful for women to lose weight.

The best way to optimize your gut flora is through your diet. A gut-healthy diet is one rich in whole, unprocessed, unsweetened foods, along with traditionally fermented or cultured foods. But before these powerful foods can work their magic in your body, you have to eliminate the damaging foods that get in their way.

The conclusions of the latest research confirm that a good place to start is by drastically reducing grains and sugar. We covered this in our very first piece of advice. Did you print out the warning and tape it to your fridge? We also need to avoid genetically engineered ingredients, processed foods, and pasteurised foods. Pasteurised foods can harm your good bacteria and sugar promotes the growth of pathogenic yeast and other fungi (not to mention fuelling cancer cells). Grains containing gluten are particularly damaging to your microflora and overall health. This would be a good time for you to review the table above that lists foods, drugs and other agents that harm your beneficial microbes so that you can take steps right now to avoid as many as possible.

And In with the Good!

Consuming naturally fermented foods is one of the best ways to optimize your microbiome.

Not only are your gut bacteria important for preventing disease, but they also play a critical role in defining your body weight and composition.

Scientific studies have revealed a positive-feedback loop between the foods you crave and the composition of your microbiome, which depends on those nutrients for survival. So, if you're craving sugar and refined carbohydrates, you may actually be feeding a voracious army of Candida! Once you've begun eliminating foods that damage your beneficial flora, start incorporating fermented foods such as sauerkraut and naturally fermented pickles for example.

Your gut bacteria - and therefore your physical and mental health - are continuously affected by your environment, and by your diet and lifestyle choices. If your microbiome is harmed and thrown out

Anti-Inflammatory Diet Your Pathway to Looking and Feeling 10 Years Younger
By Beran Parry

of balance (dysbiosis), all sorts of illnesses can result, both acute and chronic. Unfortunately, your fragile internal ecosystem is under constant assault nearly every single day.

Some of the factors posing the gravest dangers to your microbiome are outlined in the following table. You should be already familiar with some of these toxic substances from previous chapters!

- Refined sugar, especially processed high fructose corn syrup (HFCS)
- Genetically engineered (GE) foods (extremely abundant in processed foods and beverages)
- Agricultural chemicals, such as herbicides and pesticides. Glyphosate appears to be among the worst
- Conventionally-raised meats and other animal products; CAFO animals are routinely fed low-dose antibiotics and GE livestock are raised on Gluten
- Antibiotics (use only if absolutely necessary, and make sure to reseed your gut with fermented foods and/or a good probiotic supplement) NSAIDs (Nonsteroidal anti-inflammatory drugs) damage cell membranes and disrupt energy production by mitochondria)

The microbes in our gut have evolved to function as highly efficient food processors and they are directly affected by whatever we eat. When the microbiome is out of balance, we often see varying degrees of inflammation throughout the body.

The 10 years younger Diet, which is blissfully free of refined grains, flour, sugar, and processed vegetable oils supports the healthiest mixture of gut microflora. On the other hand, the typical Western diet – very high in calories from refined carbohydrates but lacking in essential nutrients – tends to have the opposite effect, contributing to a harmful imbalance in gut bacteria. This is so serious that it can lead to the development of insulin resistance, diabetes, obesity, and heart disease. An unhealthy microbiome naturally tends towards weight gain so we can see how closely our health and wellbeing is linked to the state of our intestinal flora. When the unhealthy microbes predominate in the gut, they send signals to the brain to supply more fuel in the form of refined carbohydrates, dramatically increasing the chances of you putting on more weight. As we've stated earlier in the book, taking control of your weight is only one of the benefits of creating a normal and healthy environment for your gut flora. Better health, longer life and a reduction in the risk of disease are all connected to a healthy, efficient and happy microbiome!

Anti-Inflammatory Diet Your Pathway to Looking and Feeling 10 Years Younger
By Beran Parry

Gut Biology Summary

The gut is the site of the 'second brain'

Inflammatory conditions are deeply influenced by the microbiome

Correcting intestinal flora is the key to health and weight loss

identify the toxins that harm the body and disrupt normal gut functioning

Eliminate harmful substances from daily diet to restore balance

Anti-Inflammatory Diet Your Pathway to Looking and Feeling 10 Years Younger
By Beran Parry

Anti-Inflammatory Diet Your Pathway to Looking and Feeling 10 Years Younger
By Beran Parry

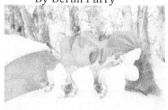

Chapter 11:

YOUR New Career

Welcome to Your brand new and exciting career! You are now Managing Director of Your. 10 YEARS YOUNGER Inc. Congratulations. It's simply the Best Job in the Whole World and now it's yours.

Your most important job from now on is to focus on making the right food choices. You don't need to weigh or measure, you don't need to count calories. Wow, I bet that sounds like a new way of dealing with the old weight loss issue, doesn't it? Just make that one decision to follow the programme under any and all circumstances, under any amount of stress and your body will do the rest.

Your only job?

The most important job in your life!

Eat the Right Food for Your Fit and Fabulous Life

Fall madly in love with your absolute best weight-loss foods - and watch them fall in love with you and your new, skinnier body

From all the information you've absorbed so far, you'll know for sure that certain food groups (like sugars, grains and dairy products) could be having a very negative impact on your health and wellbeing without you even noticing. But when you think about your present state of wellbeing, you might be wondering how much of your health - or lack of it - has been caused by the food you've been eating. Weight loss is a great example. If you've tried to lose weight but always found it a struggle, experiencing initial success but then putting the pounds back on, you know that you have to do something different. It's time to recognise that cutting down the calories isn't enough. If you're still eating the wrong foods, the problems will remain. It's time to remove the source of the problem and that's only going to happen by removing all the harmful, toxic foods from your diet.

Anti-Inflammatory Diet Your Pathway to Looking and Feeling 10 Years Younger
By Beran Parry

Say goodbye to all the psychologically unhealthy, hormone-unbalancing, gut-disrupting, inflammatory food groups and see the weight fall off. That's right. You might want to read that sentence again. It's essential to your future health. Let your body heal and recover from the years and years of weight gain and from all the other nasty effects of those nasty, toxic foods. It's time to re-programme your metabolism and flush away the inflammation.

Learn once and for all how the foods you've been eating are really affecting your health, your weight and your long term health. We've arrived at one of the most important reasons for you to follow this programme.

This is about to change your life.

Epigenetics demonstrates the vital link between the things you do and how you live to the way your body behaves, all the way down to the cellular level. This might be one of the most surprising revelations about the entire body transformation programme. I think you're going to like it because you're going to love the results.

We cannot possibly put enough emphasis on this simple fact.

Like many of the most important elements in our lives, the answers are so simple that it's too easy to blink and miss the power of this revelation.

The Skinny Delicious Transformation

Are you ready for this?

Well, take a deep breath, my friend, because this is the answer you've been waiting for.

<u>Eat. Real. Food</u>.

Eat real food.

Only eat real food.

And now you know.

Real food is unprocessed, additive free and as natural as nature intended.

Real food includes lean, organic game and poultry, line caught seafood, organic free range eggs, tons of fresh vegetables, some fruit, and plenty of good fats from fruits, oils, nuts and seeds.

Anti-Inflammatory Diet Your Pathway to Looking and Feeling 10 Years Younger
By Beran Parry

Eat foods with very few ingredients and no additives, chemicals, sugars or flavourings. Better yet, eat foods with no ingredients listed at all because then they're totally natural and unprocessed.

Don't worry, these guidelines are outlined in extensive detail in our essential life-enhancing Fifty, Fit and Fabulous Shopping list.

What to avoid if you want to be healthier, leaner, skinnier and in better shape forever.

More importantly, here's what NOT to eat. Cutting out all of these foods and drinks will help you regain your natural, healthy metabolism, reduce systemic inflammation and help you to realise exactly how these foods are truly affecting your weight, fat percentage, health, fitness and every aspect of your life.

- Sugar. It's out. It's that simple. Do not consume added sugar of any kind whether it's real or artificial. No maple syrup, honey, agave nectar, coconut sugar, Splenda, Equal, Nutrasweet, Xylitol. The only exception is Stevia, the natural sweetener that avoids the toxicity of all the other sweeteners. Start reading the labels because food companies love to use sugar in their products to cater for your sugar addiction and they use it in ways you might not recognise. Great way to sell more products. Disastrous for your health.
- Do not consume beer in any form, not even for cooking. And let's be brutal about that other global addiction - tobacco. Absolutely no tobacco products of any sort. Ever. Wine though, in moderation, is fine. Ideally you'll opt for dry wines and a small amount of spirits but NO liqueurs ever!
- Do not eat grains. This includes wheat, rye, barley, oats, corn, rice, millet, bulgur, or sprouted grains
- The very occasional exceptions are buckwheat and quinoa which are not technically grains but, unfortunately, they have many grain like qualities. The answer is to limit your consumption and always exercise moderation. Cutting out grains also includes all the ways we add wheat, corn, rice and other starches to our foods in the form of bran, wheat germ, modified starch and so on. Again, read the labels.
- Do not eat legumes, except for some occasional sprouted legumes. This includes beans of all kinds (black, red, pinto, navy, white, kidney, lima, fava, etc.), peas, chickpeas, lentils, and peanuts. No peanut butter, either. This also includes all forms of soy, soy sauce, miso, tofu, tempeh, edamame and all the many ways we sneak soy into foods (like lecithin).
- Do not eat dairy. This includes cow, goat or sheep's milk and milk products such as cream, cheese (hard or soft), kefir, yogurt (even Greek), and sour cream. Use coconut milk, coconut yoghurt and coconut cream. It's the Delicious in Skinny Delicious!

Anti-Inflammatory Diet Your Pathway to Looking and Feeling 10 Years Younger
By Beran Parry

- Do not consume carrageen an, MSG, sulphites or any additives whatsoever. If these ingredients or any E numbers appear in any form on the label of your processed food or beverage, don't even touch it!

Sounds tough, doesn't it? But that's because we've been conditioned to connect really bad food and sugary sweet flavourings with good times. We get sweets and candy as a reward during childhood and the comforting feeling gets embedded in our behaviour.

Before long we're addicted to all the things that effectively poison us. Take a look around you. Do you see much evidence of happy, healthy people in the local population? Disease incidence and obesity are ballooning. Something's radically wrong and you are one of the few, lucky ones to know exactly where the problem really lies.

Knowledge is power, my friend. Let's put this life-changing knowledge to the best possible use. Right now. You know what to do. All you have to do is make one powerful choice for health, normal weight and a tremendous increase in energy and the quality of your life and your body will do the rest.

At this stage of the programme, you might be surprised to know that we're not going to obsess too much about the weighting scales. The really important changes are taking place inside your body and your weight will improve naturally as you allow it to flush out all the toxins and reduce inflammation levels.

The Fine Print

These foods are the exceptions to the rule and the good news is they are all allowed in your new super healthy eating plan

- Certain legumes. Green beans and peas. While they're technically a legume, these are generally good for you.
- Vinegar. Most forms of vinegar, including white, apple cider, red wine, and rice, are allowed. The only exceptions are balsamic, vinegars with added sugar, or malt vinegar, which generally contains gluten.
- Salt but only low sodium or sodium-free salt. Did you know that all iodised table salt contains sugar? Sugar (often in the form of dextrose) is chemically essential to keep the potassium iodide from oxidising and being lost.

Anti-Inflammatory Diet Your Pathway to Looking and Feeling 10 Years Younger
By Beran Parry

Limitation Foods – be careful 5%
High sugar fruits – watermelon, grapes, mangoes.
Buckwheat and quinoa – it behaves like a starchy carbohydrate a bit

Clever but slightly naughty indulgences – 10%
Chocolate – organic cocoa powder,
Fried potatoes – use sweet potatoes or lots of vinegar to help with digestion,
Muffins cakes and cookies with almond and coconut flour and stevia
Nut and Seed Butters..its ok but still processed

Fats to help you burn fat – 20--%
Coconut oil, extra virgin olive oil, walnuts, macadamias and their oils, coconut products, avocados

Vegetables to fuel your system 30%
Really go to town and enjoy as many servings in as many formats as you can…raw is best, but steamed and stir fried work wonderfully well

Proteins for weight loss 35%
Fish, Turkey (chicken if you must), game and hemp seed protein are the best forms for weight loss

The 10 YEARS YOUNGER Epigenetic Shopping Guide

Being overweight is expensive in every possible way. And it costs far too much in terms of your quality of life. So it's vitally important to make healthy eating your absolute top priority and there are many of ways for you to maximize your food budget. We'll start with the top priority foods in the Skinny Delicious Diet

The next three items ALL SHARE EQUAL PRIORITY

Priority #1: Protein

Always start at the game, poultry, fish, and eggs section first because the majority of your budget should be spent on high quality animal protein.

- Prime choice:

Always look for organic and/or raised in the wild. Buy whatever's available, and learn how to cook it, if necessary. If you have room in your budget, buy extra and freeze it for later. Go for organic, free-range eggs – they're still one of the cheapest sources of good protein.

Anti-Inflammatory Diet Your Pathway to Looking and Feeling 10 Years Younger
By Beran Parry

- Alternative choice:

If you can't afford organic meat, go for game (ostrich and venison are best), fish and eggs. Chicken is still controversial because we don't know how many hormones and GMO grains are added to chickenfeed these days. Avoid beef and pork since they are too high in fat and usually contain antibiotics and hormones.

- Never:

Bypass all commercially-raised and/or processed meats (like bacon, sausage and deli meats).

- If you are against consuming animal protein for any reason, you have a great alternative in Hemp Protein Powder

Hemp protein, made from the hemp seed, is a high-fibre protein supplement that can be used to enhance total protein intake for vegans and non-vegans alike. Hemp can be considered a superior protein source due to its above-average digestibility, which also makes it ideal for athletes. When a protein is efficiently digested, it can be deployed more effectively by the body. The digestibility of any given protein is related to the concentrations of its amino acids. A study published in 2010 in the "Journal of Agricultural and Food Chemistry" tested the protein digestibility-corrected amino acid score (PDAAS) -- a rating that determines the bioavailability of a protein -- for various proteins derived from the hemp seed. The results showed that hemp seed proteins have PDAAS values greater than or equal to a variety of grains, nuts and legumes. We're big fans of hemp seed protein because it enhances the immune system and boosts energy levels as well as protecting the kidneys.

Hemp Background

Hemp is a remarkably diverse crop that can be grown for both food and non-food purposes. Hemp seed, which is used to manufacture hemp protein, is composed of approximately 45 percent oil, 35 percent protein and 10 percent carbohydrates. The hemp seed possesses many nutritional benefits, according to Agriculture and Agri-food Canada. In addition to its health benefits, hemp is very environmentally friendly, as it can be grown without the use of fungicides, herbicides and pesticides and it efficiently absorbs carbon dioxide. How many more good reasons do you need to fall in love with hemp seed protein?

Priority #2: Vegetables

Anti-Inflammatory Diet Your Pathway to Looking and Feeling 10 Years Younger
By Beran Parry

Now that you've organised your essential protein supplies, it's time to move on to the vegetables. These are the second tier of your super new plan for effective weight loss and new levels of wellbeing.

- Vegetables are very important in the epigenetic diet plan because they help the body to eliminate toxins and re-balance the microbiome. (By this we mean your gut bacteria). Local produce is the first choice and aim to eat whatever's in season as these veggies are going to be the least expensive and the most nutritious. Choose veggies that are super dense with nutrients. If you have to peel it before eating (or if you don't eat the skin), organic isn't as important. Frozen vegetables can also be an excellent budget-friendly option.
- Fruits: Buy what you can locally (and organically, if possible). If you can't get it locally then it's probably not in season, which means it's not as fresh, not as tasty, and more expensive. Frozen fruits (like berries) are superb, inexpensive alternatives. Add berries and low sugar apples to your shopping list. Bananas, peaches and pineapple should always be consumed in small quantities and we recommend that you eat sparingly grapes, mango, tropical and dried fruit especially during the three week detox phase.

Priority #3: Healthy Fats

Healthy fats make up the last items on your shopping list. Some of the healthiest fats are also the least expensive and it's always a good idea to keep a good supply of oils, nuts, and seeds at home to help in preparing your super, new skinny delicious meals.

- Canned coconut milk is delicious and provides 72 grams of fat per can. Avocados are a great, all year-round choice too when it comes to sourcing healthy fat.
- Almond milk and other nut-based milks are also recommended but always make sure there is no sugar or salt in the list of ingredients
- Almond or coconut flour make an ideal alternative for baking or for thickening sauces.
- Stock up on coconut oil, extra virgin olive oil, walnut, avocado and hazelnut oil.
- Nuts are a great source of healthy fats but you need to consume them in moderation. Nut butters often contain unnecessary additives to be careful to read the labels. Too many cheaper nuts are salted and roasted in seed or vegetable oils – a less healthy option – so always opt for the raw, natural varieties.

Additional Items

Low Sodium Salt – An Absolute Essential

Anti-Inflammatory Diet Your Pathway to Looking and Feeling 10 Years Younger
By Beran Parry

Let's start with the fact that sodium is an essential part of your daily diet. But, as many of us now know, too much sodium can be downright harmful to the body. Lower levels of sodium in the diet can really help your heart, kidneys, and all of your body systems.. The 2010 Dietary Guidelines for Americans recorded by the MayoClinic.com recommends that adults who are healthy should limit sodium to no more than 2,300 mg/day.

Sodium and Your Health

Cut down your salt intake.

The American Heart Association states that "Sodium is an element that's needed for good health. However, too much salt or too much water in your system will upset the balance." There are many benefits to following a low sodium diet. Reducing your intake of sodium, or salt, helps to reduce blood pressure and helps to prevent swelling of the extremities, such as your legs.

People who reduce their salt intake may experience an initial weight loss that is rapid, but limited. Sodium causes a person to retain water, which adds to body weight, according to Diets In Review, an online resource about healthy eating. Though someone who begins a low-sodium diet may be pleasantly surprised to see a seemingly large weight loss at first, these results typically end once the dieter returns to adding the more usual amounts of salt to their daily eating habits.

Important Considerations

Not all stevia is the same. Do try several different brands but always ensure that there are no other additives whatsoever. Stevia liquid in glycerite tends to be the best tasting!

Ways to Reduce Sodium

Salt often disguises the more subtle flavours in our food so it can be a very pleasant surprise to banish salt and discover what real food tastes like! Checking food labels will soon reveal how many daily products contain added salt. It's everywhere,. Frozen dinners, for example, can have low fat content but very high sodium levels. Using fresh or frozen vegetables can help reduce the sodium content of foods, and rinsing canned vegetables can rid them of the salt that is used in the preservation process. Using fresh or dried herbs can give meat, fish and vegetables a fabulous flavour without adding salt, fat or calories. Once you get used to less salt in your food, your taste buds come alive and reward you with a whole new sensory experience with layers of delightful subtlety that can revolutionise the eating experience forever.

The only safe sweetener for Weight Loss

Anti-Inflammatory Diet Your Pathway to Looking and Feeling 10 Years Younger
By Beran Parry

Using the highly refined extracts from the stevia leaf as a zero-calorie, 100 percent natural sweetener can help reduce your intake of sugar. Stevia is actually 300 times sweeter than regular sugar with a minimal aftertaste, yet it is suitable for sugar-sensitive people, such as diabetics. Stevia will not cause cavities and is heat-resistant enough for use in baking and cooking, according to the 2005 book by ;Dr. Gillian McKeith called Living Food for Health. Refined, simple sugars are a leading cause of obesity in the U.S., according to KidsHealth, and substituting other non-caloric sweeteners for table sugar can promote weight loss and maintenance.

The Skinny Delicious Shopping List

Items in italics – limit choice

PROTEIN

Seafood		Poultry	
Not Good:	Farm-raised	Not Good:	Factory farmed
Better:	Organic	Better:	Corn-fed
Best:	Wild-caught & sustainably fished	Best:	Organic

Game	
Not Good:	
Better:	Wild-caught
Best:	100% grass-fed & organic

Anti-Inflammatory Diet Your Pathway to Looking and Feeling 10 Years Younger
By Beran Parry

Eggs

Not Good:	Factory farmed
Better:	Organic (omega-3 enriched optional)
Best	Pastured & organic

VEGETABLES

Acorn Squash	Butternut Squash
Fennel Root	Cabbage
Artichoke	Carrots
Arugula	Cauliflower
Asparagus	Celery
Beets	Cucumber
Bell Peppers	Eggplant
Bok Choy	Garlic
Broccoli/baby broccoli	Green Beans
Brussels Sprouts	Greens (beet, mustard, turnip)

Anti-Inflammatory Diet Your Pathway to Looking and Feeling 10 Years Younger
By Beran Parry

Kale	Rhubarb
Leeks	Snow/Sugar Snap Peas
Lettuce (bibb, butter, red)	Spaghetti Squash
Mushrooms (all)	Spinach
Okra	Sprouts
Onion/Shallots	Summer Squash
Parsnips	Sweet Potato/Yams
Potatoes – smaller	Swiss Chard
Pumpkin	Tomato
Radish	Turnip
	Watercress
	Zucchini - Courgettes

Anti-Inflammatory Diet Your Pathway to Looking and Feeling 10 Years Younger
By Beran Parry

FRUITS

Apples	Exotic Fruit (star fruit, quince)
Apricots	Grapefruit
Bananas	Grapes (green/red)
Blackberries	Kiwi
Blueberries	Lemon/Lime
Cherries	Mango
Figs	Melon
Nectarines	Pomegranate
Oranges	Raspberries
Papaya	Strawberries
Peaches	Tangerines
Pears (all varieties)	Watermelon
Pineapple	NO DRIED FRUIT
Plum	

Anti-Inflammatory Diet Your Pathway to Looking and Feeling 10 Years Younger
By Beran Parry

FATS

Best: Cooking Fats	Best: Eating Fats	Sometimes: Nuts and Seeds
Coconut oil	Avocado	Almonds
Extra-Virgin Olive Oil	Cashews	Almond Butter
	Coconut Butter	Brazil Nuts
	Coconut Meat/Flakes	Pecans
	Coconut Milk (canned)	Pistachio
	Hazelnuts/Filberts	Flax Seeds
	Macadamia Nuts	Pine Nuts
	Macadamia Butter	Pumpkin Seeds
		Sesame Seeds
		Sunflower Seeds
		Seed Butters
		Walnuts

Fall in love with the best weight-loss foods

Eliminate sugars, grains and dairy products from your diet

Eat real, natural, unprocessed food

Eliminate additives

Eliminate legumes

Take charge of your body, your weight and your well being

Anti-Inflammatory Diet Your Pathway to Looking and Feeling 10 Years Younger
By Beran Parry

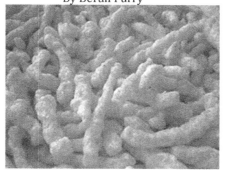

Chapter 12:

How Toxins affect weight loss and ageing

Food processing or food poisoning techniques?

The modern industrial approach to food production and processing is responsible for a ghastly range of chemicals and additives that are directly involved in producing weight gain, fat and obesity. Amongst the thousands of additives, we have bovine growth hormone and antibiotics injected into meat, poultry, and dairy products, flavour enhancers such as monosodium glutamate, artificial sweeteners such as NutraSweet (aspartame) and Splenda (sucralose). Our list also includes man-made sugars such as high fructose corn syrup, corn syrup, dextrose, sucrose, fructose, highly refined white sugar, processed molasses, processed honey, maltodextrin, etc., plus the other 15,000 plus chemicals that are routinely added to virtually every product you buy, and that includes conventionally grown fruits and vegetables.

Man-made trans-fats such as hydrogenated or partially hydrogenated oils also cause weight gain and obesity. Even standard food processing techniques such as pasteurisation, which now applies to virtually every product in a bottle or carton, homogenisation and irradiation all contribute to weight gain.

At the end of this disturbing list of toxins, poisons and health-damaging additives we have some refreshing and deeply reassuring news. Your revolutionary skinny delicious epigenetic weight control system addresses all of these issues safely and effectively and offers the fast lane out of the nightmare

Anti-Inflammatory Diet Your Pathway to Looking and Feeling 10 Years Younger
By Beran Parry

of processed food. Once you know you have the tools to make things better, you can breathe a sigh of relief and start to take action..

Poisons polluting the planet and everything that lives on it. You've probably heard a lot already about the increasing levels of toxicity in the environment. The fact is that our environment has become increasingly more toxic. Our exposure today is higher than at any point in human history.

We are exposed to more than 10,000 different forms of toxin and they are almost everywhere. They're in the air we breathe, the water we drink and wash in, our daily cleaning materials, cosmetics and, of course, our precious food supplies. If you add the daily quota of toxic chemicals we consume in the form of artificial sweeteners, flavour enhancers such as MSG, pesticides, preservatives, caffeine, over-the-counter medications, alcohol, nicotine and damaged fats, the list of daily toxic consumption could give you nightmares. But beyond the discomfort of a nightmare, these toxins are harming your body. We should also include those naturally occurring toxins produced by the body as a result of normal, essential cellular functions.

The problem is that these pesky toxins can accumulate in the body and that's when the damage occurs. It is the accumulation of these toxins that creates total havoc in the body. Yes we can process and remove many harmful substances and neutralise their influence but when we take on board more than we can handle, the body is effectively poisoned. As a result, excessive oxidative stress occurs, which in turn threatens our health by damaging our precious DNA. And as you now know, damaged DNA can lead to a long list of health problems.

Let's get this uncomfortable subject sharply into focus. Entire populations are suffering the effects of toxicity: the problems show up as a combination of headaches, fatigue, joint pain, insomnia, mood changes, weakened immune system, or other chronic issues. This total toxic overload has been implicated in: cardiovascular disease, cancer, chronic fatigue, weight loss resistance, allergies, skin conditions, asthma, mental illness, hypertension, gastritis, kidney disease and obesity. Not a happy list.

We know you like to have all the facts so let's see how toxins can even influence human metabolism.

There are five important mechanisms that are harmed by toxins:

hormone regulation,

neuro-regulatory mechanisms,

immuno-regulatory mechanisms,

Anti-Inflammatory Diet Your Pathway to Looking and Feeling 10 Years Younger
By Beran Parry

mitochondrial function,

and oxidative stress.

Toxins alter thyroid hormone metabolism and receptor function leading to a slow down in metabolic rate. Slower metabolic activity means more fat retention. It isn't difficult to see the connections between constant exposure to toxins and lots of nasty little health problems, unintended weight gain being one of the most obvious.

The Environmental Protection Agency in the U.S. has monitored human exposure to toxic environmental chemicals since 1972.

That's when they began the National Human Adipose Tissue Survey. This study measures the levels of various toxins in fat tissue extracted during autopsies and from surgical procedures. Five of what are recognised as the most toxic chemicals were found in 100% of all samples.

Toxic chemicals from industrial pollution dominated the samples, toxins that damage the liver, heart, lungs, and nervous system. Nine more chemicals were found in 91-98% of samples: benzene, toluene, ethyl benzene, DDE (a breakdown product of DDT, the pesticide banned in the US since 1972), three dioxins, and one furan. Polychlorinated biphenyls (PCBs) were found in 83% of the population.

A Michigan study found DDT in over 70% of 4 years olds, probably received through breast milk. With the spread of the global economy, we may be eating food that was picked a few days before in Guatemala, Indonesia, Africa or Asia, where there are fewer restrictions on pesticides than there are in the United States or Europe.

I don't want to put you off your lunch but many of these chemicals are stored in fat tissue, making animal products a potentially concentrated source of contamination. One hundred percent of beef in the U.S. is contaminated with DDT, as is 93% of processed cheese, hot dogs, bologna, turkey, and ice cream. Bon appetit!

But just because there are plenty of reasons to get paranoid about our food, there are plenty of healthy, life-affirming, nourishing and tasty alternatives out there.

Anti-Inflammatory Diet Your Pathway to Looking and Feeling 10 Years Younger
By Beran Parry

Toxins Summary

Pollutions and toxins are everywhere

Obesity and toxicity are closely related

The power of leptins

The thyroid connection

Cleansing and healing the body for permanent weight control

Anti-Inflammatory Diet Your Pathway to Looking and Feeling 10 Years Younger
By Beran Parry

Chapter 13:

The Exercise and 10 YEARS YOUNGER Plan

Epigenetic Exercise Myth

The Epigenetics of Exercise

Far from being written in stone, genetic expression can be altered by influences coming from outside the gene. This influence alters the operation of the gene, but does not affect the DNA blueprint itself. This process is known as epigenetics.

Toxic exposure also tends to affect genetic expression, by altering the types of proteins a particular gene will express.

In this way, your environment, diet, and general lifestyle play a significant role in your state of health and development of disease. When it comes to exercise, previous research has found that exercise can induce *immediate* changes in the methylation patterns of genes found in your muscle cells.

Several of the genes affected by an acute bout of exercise are genes involved in fat metabolism. Specifically, the study suggests that when you exercise, your body almost immediately experiences genetic activation that increases the production of fat-busting proteins.

Quite clearly, exercise in all its forms tends to have a positive effect. It has the power to affect your entire body, and your overall state of health. Its beneficial impact on your insulin response (normalizing your glucose and insulin levels by optimizing insulin receptor sensitivity) is among the most important benefits of exercise, as insulin resistance is a factor in most chronic disease.

The Many Biological Effects of Exercise

Getting back to the effects of exercise in general, a number of biological effects occur when you work out. This includes changes in your:
- **Muscles**, which use glucose and ATP for contraction and movement. To create more ATP, your body needs extra oxygen, so breathing increases and your heart starts pumping more blood to your muscles. Without sufficient oxygen, lactic acid will form instead. Tiny tears in your muscles make them grow bigger and stronger as they heal.

Anti-Inflammatory Diet Your Pathway to Looking and Feeling 10 Years Younger
By Beran Parry

- **Lungs**. As your muscles call for more oxygen (as much as 15 times more oxygen than when you're at rest), your breathing rate increases. Once the muscles surrounding your lungs cannot move any faster, you have reached what's called your VO2 max your maximum capacity of oxygen use. The higher your VO2 max, the fitter you are.

- **Heart**. As mentioned, your heart rate increases with physical activity to supply more oxygenated blood to your muscles. The fitter you are, the more efficiently your heart can do this, allowing you to work out longer and harder. As a side effect, this increased efficiency will also reduce your *resting* heart rate. Your blood pressure will also decrease as a result of new blood vessels forming.

- **Joints and bones**, as exercise can place as much as five or six times more than your body weight on them. Peak bone mass is achieved in adulthood and then begins a slow decline, but exercise can help you to maintain healthy bone mass as you get older. Weight-bearing exercise is actually one of the most effective remedies against osteoporosis, as your bones are very porous and soft, and as you get older your bones can easily become less dense and hence, more brittle -- especially if you are inactive.

Exercise Is Important for Optimal Brain Health, Too

Genetic changes occur here, too. The increased blood flow adapts your brain to turn different genes on or off, and many of these changes help protect against diseases such as Alzheimers and Parkinsons. A number of neurotransmitters are also triggered, such as endorphins, serotonin, dopamine, glutamate, and GABA. Some of these are well-known for their role in mood control. Not surprisingly, exercise is one of the most effective prevention and treatment strategies for depression. Exercise Leverages Other Healthy Lifestyle Changes

While diet accounts for about 80 percent of the health benefits you get from a healthy lifestyle, exercise is the ultimate leveraging agent that kicks all those benefits up a notch. The earlier you begin and the more consistent you are, the greater your long-term rewards, but its never too late to start. Even seniors can improve their physical and mental health.

Its strongly recommend to avoid sitting as much as possible, and making it a point to walk more every day. A fitness tracker can be very helpful for this. I suggest aiming for 7,000 to 10,000 steps per day, *in addition to* your regular fitness regimen, not in lieu of it. The research is clearly showing that prolonged sitting is an independent risk factor for chronic disease and increases your mortality risk from *all* causes. So standing up more and engaging in non-exercise movement as much as possible is just as important for optimal health as having a regular fitness regimen.

Anti-Inflammatory Diet Your Pathway to Looking and Feeling 10 Years Younger
By Beran Parry

One of the great myths about weight loss is that all you have to do is burn more calories and everything will be absolutely fine. Clearly, from all the information we've studied and absorbed so far, we know this cannot be the whole story.

We know for a fact that people can lose weight by burning more calories. No question.

The problem is that it's rarely a permanent loss. As soon as you take a break from the routine, the pounds pile back on. And we're committed to a permanent and healthy weight adjustment that will benefit every aspect of your life. So let's remind ourselves that if we're going to take control of our weight, we need to change our metabolism. If we can encourage our metabolism to speed up, we'll burn our food more efficiently and encourage our bodies to burn fat.

Adding exercise to our routine can certainly help to speed up the weight loss programme but we're encouraging you to exercise because it really can improve the overall quality of your life. We want you to be fitter, stronger, leaner, more flexible and happier in the way your body works. Does that sound like a good idea? Do you want to live in a body that works the way Nature intended? It's a lot more fun than being trapped in an overweight, physically uncomfortable body that lacks the energy and stamina to enjoy life to the full.

When it comes to exercise, we're truly spoiled for choice. It seems that every time we turn on the TV there's a super-fit girl or boy bouncing up and down with the latest fitness fad, screaming at us to join the craze. But fitness is not about fashion. It isn't about gadgets and it isn't about trying to look like someone else. It's about feeling great and making the body as efficient as nature intended. Yes, we have to move the body to make it fitter but using exercise intelligently will serve our purposes better than blindly following the latest exercise in television fitness marketing.

The first question to raise in our quest for intelligent exercise is "What kind of exercise will help me lose excess fat and weight most efficiently?" The short answer, perhaps not surprisingly, is the kind of exercise that burns the most calories. But we need to burn calories in the most efficient manner possible for the longest period of time whilst encouraging an increase in metabolic rate. OK. Not such a short answer but even a simple question can offer important insights into what we're really seeking in terms of safe, intelligent exercise.

There is a common consensus that cardiovascular workouts are the best in terms of straightforward calorie burning but there is a growing realisation that interval workouts, where we switch between short bursts of high intensity effort followed by brief periods of less intense exercise, are one of the best ways to turn up the fat-burning mechanism. Interval training can raise your metabolic rate for up to four hours after a session, meaning you'll burn more calories even after the workout is over.

Anti-Inflammatory Diet Your Pathway to Looking and Feeling 10 Years Younger
By Beran Parry

Easy? Well before you jump into your exercise shorts and slip on the Spandex leotard, we need to recognise that too many intense cardio sessions can harm your body, causing burn out, leaving you tired, low in energy, suffering strained joints and muscles and too exhausted to keep up the exercise programme. Less is sometimes more. Try using the higher intensity interval approach a couple of days a week and substitute a less intense endurance session for your other workouts. Endurance training means exercising at an intensity where you can still talk without getting breathless. This combination gives the body time to recover, reduces strain whilst still promoting a more efficient metabolism. And you'll probably enjoy it more too.

Muscle, my friend. You were probably wondering about muscles, weren't you? You'll definitely need more metabolically active lean muscle mass to give your body new strength, shape and definition while you continue to reveal the skinnier new you. Light resistance exercises will help. Using lighter weights will help you use whole body without risk of strain or injury Lighter weights mean more repetitions and more reps will give you the lean definition that is a sure sign of a fit and healthy body.

The real challenge is getting started, taking the first step and then committing to a programme of movement and exercise. That's why it's helpful to recognise the importance of enjoying the exercise as much as possible. Find alternatives to the dreaded treadmill. Join group classes that focus on high energy movement. Take Pilates classes every week or follow a Pilates video with an excellent teacher. The body positively thrives on new and different movements so yoga and Pilates are fantastic ways to develop a stronger, more flexible body. An active yoga class, for example, that keeps your heart rate elevated can count as a cardio session and a Pilates class that incorporates added resistance from bands or weights can count as strength training.

Finally, don't forget that it's really easy to eat back all the calories you burned off at the gym in just a few unplanned minutes of pure self-indulgence. So for permanent weight loss success, combine your workouts with our Skinny Delicious Epigenetic Diet. That's an unbeatable combination for health, fitness and total wellbeing.

Anti-Inflammatory Diet Your Pathway to Looking and Feeling 10 Years Younger
By Beran Parry

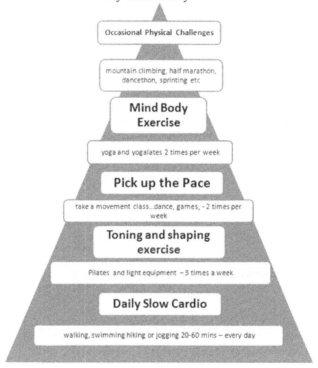

Here are the Skinny Delicious Intelligent Exercise Choices that have proved effective time and time again!

Walking your way to weight loss? Yes! It absolutely helps.

1. Walking

Walking really is an ideal exercise for weight loss even if your eyebrows just shot up in surprise! Walking really works. But it's something you have to do every single day. You don't need special equipment, you don't need special clothes, you don't even need a gym membership to do it. Just you and a pair of comfortable shoes. It's a low-impact exercise too, which reduces strain on your knees, feet and hips.

For those with obesity and heart disease, walking is an effective, low-intensity weight-loss activity that can lead to better overall health, as well as better mental wellbeing. Depending on how much you weigh, walking at a pace of four miles per hour will burn between 5 and 8 calories every minute, or between 225 and 360 calories for a 45-minute stroll. If you're interested in the maths, walking every day at this pace for 45 minutes can mean losing up to a pound a week without changing any other habits. That's every week and the accumulative effect can be truly dramatic.

So put on your walking shoes, turn up the headphones and go for a brisk stroll through the neighbourhood. If you live close to where you work or shop, make walking your primary mode of transportation and watch the excess weight slip away. Don't let the weather get in the way of your daily walk. When the weather's bad, walk indoors or take your stroll on a treadmill.

There's a lot to be said for breathing fresh air too so, if the opportunity presents itself, experience the joy of taking a walk in the woods or in the countryside. It's a good idea to take water with you too, keeping the body properly hydrated. If you aren't used to walking, take your time.

Start gently. Don't push yourself too much. Patience is a key to good exercise routines and building up your capacity to do more should leave you feeling motivated to extend your range until you can walk comfortably for as long as you wish. That in itself can mark a significant achievement and boost your confidence in your increasing levels of fitness.

Splish splash! Come on in, the water's lovely!

2. Swimming

Swimming is such a fun way to enjoy your exercise. It's another great way to share the benefits of physical exercise and include the family as well. The great news is that this exercise works. It's really effective for weight loss and for toning. When we swim, we use all the major muscle groups, including your abdominals and back muscles, your arms, legs, hips and glutes. It's a great way of enhancing the effects of other exercises, like running and walking, or it can be your preferred form of fitness. It's also widely recognised that swimming is ideal during pregnancy, especially during the last trimester, but it's often forgotten that it's a perfect way to exercise for obese individuals and for arthritis sufferers. Water supports ninety percent of the body's weight yet provides twelve times the resistance of air so moving or swimming in the pool is a perfect way to strengthen and tone the body whilst burning calories.

Swimming has long been used as an effective tool for building stamina so you can look forward to getting fitter and building healthy reserves of energy whilst having fun in the water. Whether you're walking from side to side in the shallow end or swimming lengths, the pool is a perfect place to measure your progress. Just add an extra width or length every week and you'll be amazed how quickly your fitness levels start to climb.

Don't be square. Round is much more fun!

3. Elliptical Training

A fantastic alternative to the dreaded treadmill is the elliptical trainer, regarded by many as the better way to work out at home or at the gym. The main advantage over the conventional treadmill is that the elliptical trainer provides a low impact cardio workout that reduces strain on the key, load-bearing joints of the body. It's an ideal piece of equipment for burning calories and boosting the metabolism. Elliptical trainers have moving handles which encourage you to move your arms and give you the benefit of an upper body workout. You can select an appropriate level of resistance and intensity to match your growing levels of strength and fitness and you can expect to burn a respectable 600 calories an hour.

When you're overweight, running places enormous strain on your joints and the combination of poor posture, inadequate muscle strength and poor lumbar support is a recipe for pain and injury. The elliptical trainer is an ideal machine for allowing gentle, safe and controlled movement without stressing hips, knees and ankles. The elliptical movement that the equipment is named for reduces back strain and opens up the possibility of effective and risk free weight reduction.

As with swimming, you can increase the speed or intensity of the workout every week and build up your stamina, strength and fitness gently, carefully and effectively as the excess pounds fall away.

Anti-Inflammatory Diet Your Pathway to Looking and Feeling 10 Years Younger
By Beran Parry

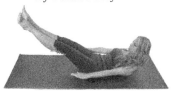

Not just for supermodels! Pilates really is for everyone. And that includes you!

4. Pilates

As a Pilates Master Teacher and Yoga Teacher, I can vouch for the fact that Pilates especially contributes to weight loss – and so does yoga – but this indirectly as explained later on in the chapter...but look at the change in shape of my body and that is all you need to see if you are looking at getting into your best shape!

Pilates is deservedly famous for creating longer, leaner, fitter bodies. The Pilates method promotes weight loss and a leaner, more muscular appearance. But how does it work?

The precisely positioned exercise burn calories. How many calories you burn obviously depends on your body type and the level of effort.

Creating lean muscle mass, as Pilates does, is one of the best ways to increase your calorie-burning potential.

Pilates tones and shapes the whole body.

Sample some Pilates mat exercises:

One of the best ways to look and feel thinner is to have beautiful posture. Pilates creates a leaner look by emphasizing both length and better, healthier bodily alignment.

Pilates promotes deep and efficient respiration, which is essential for calorie burning and tissue regeneration.

Engaging in an exercise program, like Pilates, promotes self-esteem and heightened lifestyle consciousness. Both are associated with weight loss.

Anti-Inflammatory Diet Your Pathway to Looking and Feeling 10 Years Younger
By Beran Parry

One of the most frequently asked questions about Pilates is: Will Pilates help me lose weight? The short answer is yes, Pilates is supportive but not the cause of weight loss. In many cases just beginning a Pilates class, or a home routine, is enough to jump start weight loss. However, as time goes by you may find that your body becomes accustomed to your workout level. Then, you will need to increase the intensity of your workout enough to help you continue to burn extra calories. Here are some ideas to help you ramp up your workout:

If you take a Pilates class regularly, talk to your instructor and find out if it is possible to move the class along a little more quickly. Sometimes a class needs to take that step. On the other hand, it may be that some members of your class are not ready to increase the pace of their workouts and you will have to graduate yourself to a more advanced class.

If you workout at home, it is a good idea to have a routine or two that you know quite well. That way you can focus on the breath and flow of the workout and not have to pause to review the exercise instructions or sequence.

Another great way to get a weight loss workout at home is to expand your Pilates DVD collection. Look for workouts that push your current level or add a new challenge like the magic circle, fitness band, or exercise ball. There are also a number of excellent Pilates based DVDs specifically oriented toward weight loss. As a Pilates Master Trainer I will be happy to give you a personal recommendation for good quality Pilates DVD's. Contact me at beranparry@gmail.com

Fully Commit to Each Exercise

Even if you can't move through a routine rapidly, do make sure that you get the most out of each exercise. Stretch to your fullest length at every opportunity, go for the extra scoop of the abs, breathe deeply, be precise, move with control and grace. This kind of fully engaged attitude is very much in keeping with what Joseph Pilates taught, and increases the exertion level (read weight loss potential) of your workout tremendously.

Add Equipment

Adding equipment , or different equipment, to your workout will help build muscle and strength by giving your body new challenges. Remember, muscle burns a lot of fat. If you go to a studio to workout, you could move from the mat to the reformer. If you have been using the reformer, take a chance and sign up for a class that includes a new piece of equipment, like the wunda chair or ladder barrel.

At home, smaller types of Pilates equipment such as magic circles, exercise balls and fitness bands can add the extra challenge. They also help keep your workouts interesting.

Anti-Inflammatory Diet Your Pathway to Looking and Feeling 10 Years Younger
By Beran Parry

Use Less Resistance

Now here is a Pilates trick that is not used by many other fitness systems: If you are working out with Pilates resistance equipment, decrease the resistance level. This seems counter intuitive, but the instability that less resistance creates provides a significant challenge to the muscles as they attempt to maintain control and balance, especially the core muscles. This technique works very well on the reformer where you can use lighter springs, but you can apply the same principle to a lighter resistance magic circle or fitness band. You may be surprised at the level of intensity that instability can add to your workout, especially as you work to maintain precision and control during both the exertion and the release phase of an exercise, as we do in Pilates.

Anti-Inflammatory Diet Your Pathway to Looking and Feeling 10 Years Younger
By Beran Parry

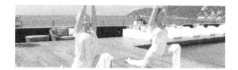

Will Doing Yoga Help Me Lose Weight?

5. Yoga

Doing yoga regularly offers many benefits, including making you feel better about your body as you become stronger and more flexible, toning your muscles, reducing stress, and improving your mental and physical well-being. But will it help you lose weight? Practicing any type of yoga will build strength, but studies show that yoga does not raise your heart rate enough to make it the only form of exercise you need to shed pounds.

In order to lose weight, you must eat correctly and burn calories by doing exercise that raises your heart rate on a regular basis. More vigorous yoga styles can provide a better workout than gentle yoga, but if weight loss is your primary goal, you will want to combine yoga with running, walking, or other aerobic exercise.

How Yoga Can Help

Yoga can still help you lose weight by bringing you to a better in tune with your body, improving your self-image and sense of well-being, and encouraging a healthy lifestyle.

If you are just starting to do yoga , are very overweight , or are quite out of shape, always choose a beginner-level class. To minimize the risk of injury, make sure find good teachers and listen to your body first and foremost.

What Kinds of Yoga Are the Most Vigorous?

The most athletic yoga styles fall in the vinyasa or flow yoga category. These styles usually start with a fast-paced series of poses called sun salutations, followed by a flow of standing poses which will keep you moving. Once you are warmed up, deeper stretches and backbends are introduced. Vinyasa includes many popular, sweaty yoga styles, such as:

Ashtanga:

Ashtanga yoga is a very vigorous style of practice and its practitioners are among the most dedicated of yogis. Beginners are often encouraged to sign up for a series of classes, which will help with motivation.

Power Yoga:

Power yoga is extremely popular at gyms and health clubs, though it is widely available at dedicated yoga studios as well. Power yoga is based on building the heat and intensity of Ashtanga while dispensing with fixed series of poses.

Hot Yoga:

Vinyasa yoga done in a hot room ups the ante by guaranteeing you'll sweat buckets. Be aware that Bikram and hot yoga are not synonymous. Bikram is a pioneering style of hot yoga, which includes a set series of poses and, indeed, a script developed by founder Bikram Choudhury. These days, there are many other styles of hot yoga that make use of the hot room but not the Bikram series.

Yoga Workouts at Home

Keep yourself exercising by doing yoga at home on the days you can't make a class. Follow along with a video if you are new to yoga. When you are ready to plan your own workouts, use these yoga sequencing ideas to help you come up with yoga sessions of varying lengths that will fit your schedule. To maximize yoga's benefits, it's great to do a little bit each day.

Your Skinny Delicious Exercise Plan and Log

Keeping an exercise log helps you stay motivated, track progress, and plan improvements. This becomes even more relevant when you have a goal like weight loss.

Skinny Delicious Exercise Planner and Workbook

Anti-Inflammatory Diet Your Pathway to Looking and Feeling 10 Years Younger
By Beran Parry

	Monday	Tuesday	Wednesday	Thursday	Friday	Saturday	Sunday
AM	walking 20-60 minutes or a slow jog or swimming	walking 20-60 minutes or a slow jog elliptical or cycling training or take a fun dance or movement class	walking 20-60 minutes or a slow jog or swimming	walking 20-60 minutes or a slow jog elliptical or cycling training or take a fun dance or movement class	walking 20-60 minutes or a slow jog or swimming	walking 20-60 minutes or a slow jog elliptical or cycling training or take a fun dance or movement class	walking 20-60 minutes or a slow jog
PM	Pilates	yoga	Pilates	yoga	Pilates		
Eve	10-60 minutes meditation	10-60 minutes meditation	10-60 minutes meditation	10-60 minutes meditation	10-60 minutes meditation	10-60 minutes meditation	10-60 minutes meditation

Workout More Frequently

Working out more often is an obvious choice for weight loss and it can work like a charm. After all, the more opportunity you take to increase your respiration, build strength, and tone your muscles, the more weight you can lose and the trimmer you will appear.

Anti-Inflammatory Diet Your Pathway to Looking and Feeling 10 Years Younger
By Beran Parry

Exercise Summary

Check out a selection of exercises that are best for weight loss

The smart way to exercise is best

Walking your way to health – a fabulous daily habit!

Swimming as a safe alternative – or choose something unusual

Use Pilates to shape your body!

Boost your programme with Yoga

Anti-Inflammatory Diet Your Pathway to Looking and Feeling 10 Years Younger
By Beran Parry

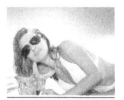

Chapter 14:

Your anti-ageing and weight loss helpers! Vitamin D and Magnesium

Now that you've taken the most important steps possible to take total control of your weight and give your body the best possible opportunity to feel simply amazing, it's time to introduce you to a select group of helpers that can make your programme even more effective. We're going to start with Vitamin D, the famous sunshine vitamin. Now, as you might have guessed by now, we love sharing the results of cutting edge medical and scientific research. So when we looked at the conclusions of over 3,000 independent clinical studies that have been carried out all over the world in the last year alone, we were not surprised to learn that good old Vitamin D has now been recognised as the superstar in the weight loss supplement industry.

Vitamin D and Weight Loss

Vitamin D is produced by the body when it's exposed to sunlight. It's a naturally occurring substance and it can also be acquired through diet or supplements. The great news is that it increases the metabolic energy of fat cells which encourages faster weight loss. Surprised? Happy to have another potent asset to help you move those excess pounds and keep you trimmer, fitter and healthier? Not only does it speed up metabolic rates for fat cells but it helps to eliminate toxins too. Now that's another great reason to ensure healthy levels of Vitamin D in your body.

One surprising insight that has emerged from the research is that both muscle and fat may well act in a similar way when it comes to storing vitamin D for future use.

New research using mathematical models has shown that a heavily muscled man and an obese man who weigh exactly the same would need the same amount of vitamin D. The key to determining

Anti-Inflammatory Diet Your Pathway to Looking and Feeling 10 Years Younger
By Beran Parry

how much vitamin D is appropriate for an individual would seem to be connected to body weight rather than body fat. The research is fresh so this important revelation has not been widely appreciated by most experts.

If you're overweight you're more likely to need more vitamin D than a thinner person. This new rule also applies to people with higher body weights even when it's a result of muscle mass.

Your best source for this vitamin is daily exposure to the sun, without sunblock on your skin, until your skin turns the lightest shade of pink. Too much sun is as bad as too little so don't be tempted to overdose on anything and that includes sunshine. Getting healthy exposure to the sun isn't always possible due to seasonal changes and the simple fact of where you live but moderate exposure is the ideal to aim for as it will optimize your vitamin D levels naturally.

To use the sun to maximize your vitamin D production and minimize your risk of skin damage, the middle of the day (roughly between 10:00 a.m. and 2:00 p.m.) is the best and safest time. During this UVB-intense period you will need the shortest sun exposure time to produce the most vitamin D.

If getting out into the sunshine isn't possible, you might consider using one of the safer tanning beds. These use electronic rather than magnetic ballasts and this avoids unnecessary EMF exposure. Safe tanning beds produce less of the dangerous UVA than sunlight, while unsafe ones have more UVA than sunlight. If neither of these options are available to you, then you should take an oral vitamin D3 supplement and this is where the dosage becomes important.

What's the Correct Dose of Vitamin D?

Based on research published by GrassrootsHealth from the D*Action study, the average adult needs to take 8,000 IU's of vitamin D per day in order to elevate his or her levels above 40 ng/ml. This is considered to be the minimum requirement necessary for disease prevention. Ideally, you'll want your levels to be between 50-70 ng/ml. As Carole Baggerly, director and founder of GrassrootsHealth, noted:

"We just published our very first paper. We have about 10 people in this study now that are taking 50,000 IU a day and they're not reaching a potential toxicity level of 200 ng/ml. It should be noted, however, that this is not a recommended intake level. The study reported data on about over 3,500 people. ... One very significant thing shown by this research was that even with taking the supplement, the curve for the increase in the vitamin D level is not linear. It is curvilinear and it flattens, which is why it's even hard to get toxic with a supplement."

This means that even if you do not monitor your vitamin D levels on a regular basis, there is very little risk of taking too much. There is evidence that the safety of vitamin D is dependent on vitamin K, and that vitamin D toxicity (although very rare with the D3 form) is actually aggravated by vitamin K2 deficiency. So if you take oral vitamin D, ideally you should take vitamin K2 as well or use organic fermented foods that are high in vitamin K2, as you need about 150 mcg per day.

It must be said that it is challenging to work out precisely how much vitamin D your body produces naturally and then calculate how much you might need in supplement form. Most people are deficient in Vitamin D and the best way to correct this imbalance is to consult your doctor, take the 25 OH D blood test and then either increase your exposure to sunlight or request supplements with a dose somewhere in the range of 5,000-40,000 IU. Follow up tests should be done to check your new Vitamin D levels after a few months of taking the recommended supplements.

The latest clinical data concerning the benefits of healthy Vitamin D levels reveal that this essential chemical does a lot more than help with weight issues. It's got an impressive list of advantages for everyone:

- targets belly fat first
- turns body into fat burning mode instead of fat storing mode
- lowers high blood pressure
- helps form stronger bones to fight osteoporosis
- helps protect against different cancers
- boosts natural immune system
- reduces inflammation & joint stiffness
- influences the important hormone leptin

Calcium and the Link to Vitamin D

As you can see from the list above, there are many health benefits associated with having sufficient Vitamin D in the body. When the body experiences a lack of calcium, it is usually due to a vitamin D deficiency. This triggers the body to increase its production of synthase, a fatty acid enzyme that turns calories into fat. A calcium deficiency will cause the body to increase its synthase production by up to 500%, which may explain a further cause of obesity. When vitamin D supplements are combined with sunlight, calcium, and a low-calorie diet, it helps the body to regulate blood sugar levels, digest food properly and, for those who are interested in losing the excess pounds, it also promotes weight loss.

Recommended Intake of Vitamin D

The recommended daily intake of vitamin D should be between 400 and 600 IU. However, current research has suggested that a higher dosage would be more therapeutic. In order to improve health and heal the body, the body needs approximately 4,000 and 10,000 IU of vitamin D per day. Depending

Anti-Inflammatory Diet Your Pathway to Looking and Feeling 10 Years Younger
By Beran Parry

on skin tone, the body will need 10 to 20 minutes of sun every day to produce 10,000 IU of vitamin D. When the sun is not a viable option, it is best to supplement your diet with a vitamin D supplement.

2. Magnesium and Weight Loss

Obesity. Is it really connected to your epigenetic behaviour?

The popular view in the media has constantly repeated the myth that obesity is somehow inherited. People have looked at their obese relatives, sighed sadly over their bulging stomachs and resigned themselves to the apparent injustice of their bad genes. But it just isn't that simple. Oh, no. If you take a mouse with an obesity gene and deprive it of B vitamins, the obesity will be expressed. The mouse gets chubby. But if it receives plenty of B vitamins, the obese gene stays in neutral and our little mouse stays thin. The process of metabolising B vitamins is called methylation and magnesium is one of the most important elements in this process.

Magnesium plays a crucial role in many aspects of the body's health but here are some of the most relevant examples

1. Magnesium helps the body to digest, absorb, and process proteins, fats, and carbohydrates.
2. Magnesium is an essential chemical to allow insulin to open cell membranes for glucose.
3. Magnesium helps prevent obesity genes from expressing themselves.

Magnesium and THE WEIGHT CONNECTION

Magnesium and the B complex vitamins are important for helping to access the energy that's contained within our food. They're responsible for switching on enzymes that control digestion, nutrient absorption and the way we process proteins, fats, and carbohydrates. When our bodies don't get enough of these essential nutrients, we can experience a surprising range of negative consequences. Some of the unexpected consequences include hypoglycaemia, anxiety, depression and even our old friend, obesity.

The fact is that amidst an extraordinary array of foods and an incredible choice of what and how much to eat, we are often starved of essential nutrients. There is a fascinating research project that has identified the connection between our food cravings for foods and the way our bodies lack those essential nutrients.

Processed foods that lack the essential nutritional content that supports healthy metabolism are effectively empty calories. They only serve to add unhealthy weight to the body without contributing to the body's total nutritional requirements. So, as a result, you're often really hungry. So you keep eating.

Anti-Inflammatory Diet Your Pathway to Looking and Feeling 10 Years Younger
By Beran Parry

But you're still hungry and your body's packing on the extra weight but in reality you're starved of good nutrition.

The study suggested that changing to a healthy diet can re-set the brain's triggers for high fat, high calorie food and create a much healthier response to food choices that avoids over-eating and focuses on a naturally low-fat, high energy diet. You just know that's going to help to keep the unwanted weight off and introduce you to a whole new world of feeling great.

Magnesium also produces the metabolic reaction that instructs insulin to allow the transfer of energy-providing glucose into our cells. If the body doesn't have enough magnesium to fulfil this important role, both insulin and glucose levels increase. The excess glucose is converted into fat and this obviously contributes to obesity problems. Having excess insulin also raises the risk of diabetes.

Is stress connected to weight gain? Oh yes it is. But we have the answer!

The powerful connection between stress and obesity has long been understood. When our bodies are stressed, we produce more of the chemical cortisol and the cortisol effectively forces a metabolic reversal that makes weight loss almost impossible. The great news is that our good friend and helper, magnesium, can effectively neutralise these undesirable effects of stress.

ABDOMINAL Fat - Is a corset the only answer? No!!

Gaining weight around your middle is strongly related to magnesium deficiency and an inability to properly utilise insulin. This is when we run the risk of encountering Syndrome X. You only need a tape measure to diagnose a predisposition to Syndrome X. If you have a waist size above 40 inches in men and above 35 in women then you're at risk. In their book The Magnesium Factor, authors Mildred Seelig, M.D., and Andrea Rosanoff, Ph.D., refer to research that demonstrates over half the insulin in the bloodstream is directed at abdominal tissue. They suggest that as more and more insulin is produced to deal with a high-sugar diet, abdominal size increases mainly to process the extra insulin.

Magnesium and SYNDROME X

The term "syndrome X" refers to a set of conditions that are really the product of long-standing nutritional deficiency, especially magnesium deficiency. Syndrome X is simply the result of starving the body of those essential nutrients. The long list of problems includes high cholesterol, hypertension and obesity. It also includes elevated triglycerides and high levels of uric acid. High triglycerides are usually found when cholesterol levels are too high but it happens most often with people who consume a daily high-sugar diet and that includes fizzy drinks, cakes, biscuits, candy and pastries. Syndrome X is a description of what happens when we eat badly.

Anti-Inflammatory Diet Your Pathway to Looking and Feeling 10 Years Younger
By Beran Parry

Vitamins and minerals are the driving forces that produce our metabolism. Without them, we get problems. So, the first step in treating non-specific symptoms is to consider diet and dietary supplements, not drugs. It is also important to note that many of the diets that people adopt to lose weight are often deficient in the vital ingredient that can make such an important contribution to weight control - magnesium.

We mentioned above that magnesium is an essential part of the process that allows insulin to play its part in the way that glucose is transferred into our cells. The cells need that energy to function normally so, if there isn't enough magnesium, the cells can't absorb the glucose and this is what follows:

1. Glucose levels become elevated.
2. Glucose is stored as fat and leads to obesity.
3. Elevated glucose leads to diabetes.
4. Obesity puts a strain on the heart.
5. Excess glucose becomes attached to certain proteins (glycated), leading to kidney damage, neuropathy, blindness, and other diabetic complications.
6. Insulin-resistant cells don't allow magnesium into the cells.
7. Further magnesium deficiency leads to hypertension.
8. Magnesium deficiency leads to cholesterol build-up and both these conditions are implicated in heart disease.

Syndrome X, according to Dr. Gerald Reaven, the individual who coined the term, may be responsible for a large percentage of the heart and artery disease that occurs today. Unquestionably, magnesium deficiency is a major factor in the origins of each of its signs and symptoms, from elevated triglycerides and obesity to disturbed insulin metabolism.

INSULIN RESISTANCE

Food. Food. Glorious Food.

We've made lots of references and observations about food. Well, it's one of the keys to truly great weight management. It's time now to take a closer look at the way that specific foods can make you gain unwanted weight at an alarming rate and stack the fat around your belly.

Insulin is a very powerful hormone and, as you might expect, it can produce very powerful reactions in humans. You've probably seen news items and articles referring to the glycemic index. Foods that feature at the top of this index are a cause of massive increases in insulin secretion and this produces intense cravings, hunger and an increase in fat production. Foods that score high on the glycemic index are a disaster for healthy weight control and a menace to good health. There's a great deal of debate about saturated or unsaturated fats. All of these components have some level of

Anti-Inflammatory Diet Your Pathway to Looking and Feeling 10 Years Younger
By Beran Parry

importance. However, nutritionists and doctors virtually never mention the most important and significant components of food which can lead to weight gain and obesity. We need to lift the lid right now on food processing techniques

We've identified a key role that insulin plays in the body: it opens up sites on cell membranes to allow the flow of glucose, a cell's source of energy. Cells that no longer respond to the signals from insulin and refuse the entry of glucose are called insulin-resistant. As a result, blood glucose levels rise and the body produces more and more insulin. Glucose and insulin are pumped around the body, causing tissue damage that results in further depletion of magnesium, an increased risk of heart disease and the likelihood of adult onset diabetes.

So, get your weight loss cure today. Start taking magnesium, soak in Epsom Bath Salts or spray it on your body and watch the weight drop off. Sometimes it really is the simplest things that can make the most dramatic difference. In this case, we're highlighting magnesium as one of the best allies we can recruit to our weight control cause.

Anti-Inflammatory Diet Your Pathway to Looking and Feeling 10 Years Younger
By Beran Parry

Helpers - Summary

The power of sunshine and the Vitamin D connection

Magnesium and weight loss

Syndrome X

Insulin resistance

Relieving health issues with smart nutrition

Disclaimer:

The information you have read in this chapter needs to be matched with your current medical status to determine how to use these fantastic weight loss aids safely and effectively. Please consult with a Functional Medicine Specialist in order to take these supplements safely. I will be happy to recommend a suitable professional in your area. Just contact me on beranparry@gmail.com

Anti-Inflammatory Diet Your Pathway to Looking and Feeling 10 Years Younger
By Beran Parry

Chapter 15:

10 YEARS YOUNGER DAILY FOOD AND DINING OUT GUIDE

Your Personal Guide to a Skinnier, New You is full of the latest research on how your body really works. We've armed and prepared you with the science, the knowledge and the facts about intelligent, effective weight control and now we want to expand your knowledge further by sharing a great list of things that you can eat and enjoy plus a list of the unhelpful things that you really cannot afford to have in your diet if you plan to control your weight and discover the real meaning of total health. You're going to be a great detective and find all the clues to what you're really eating by reading the labels on your food.

Sugar, my little sweetie, is always off the menu. Just because the amount listed is very small, it's still sugar and you have to look for every form of sweetener, real or artificial, because if it's on the label it just isn't going into your mouth. Sugar is out. Gone. Adios, amigo. Forever.

Almond Flour. "You can make flour from almonds?" Yes you can and you can eat it. People are discovering the benefits of coconut flour too because these flours do not come from grains. That makes them much safer alternatives to the traditional flour that contains inflammatory-provoking glutens. It's even possible to make almond milk too but the commercially produced variety usually contains sweeteners so gets disqualified before you even open the carton. If in doubt, it's better to make your own almond milk and that way you can absolutely control the purity of the ingredients. The controversial use of almond flour is to use it as a substitute for baking bread, biscuits or anything else where we would previously have used regular flour. In cleansing the body, it might not be appropriate to use almond or coconut flour for baking. Sorry.

Bacon is incredibly popular because it tastes so good. One of the reasons for that great flavour is that the meat processors often add sugar as a preservative and flavour enhancer. Sourcing hormone-free and antibiotic-free meat is a real challenge so bacon is definitely off the menu.

Bean sprouts have been a staple of the vegetarian diet since records began but it's the plant that is good to eat, not the seeds. The beans contain compounds that are difficult for humans to digest successfully. So it's a resounding yes to the sprouts and no to the beans themselves.

Bread. You're not serious, are you? Did you expect a green light for bread? Sorry, folks. It's definitely a no. Make that a capital N-O just to be certain. If you miss the old demon slice of toxicity, try using almond flour, sweet potato flour or flaxseed flour as your new basic ingredient for making a dramatically healthier alternative to grain-based bread.

Anti-Inflammatory Diet Your Pathway to Looking and Feeling 10 Years Younger
By Beran Parry

Buckwheat might surprise you because it's long been associated with the image of a healthy diet. Buckwheat though is a pseudo cereal. Technically speaking, it isn't a grain but it still causes similar problems to all the grains we're eliminating from our daily diet. So buckwheat goes onto the No No pile.

Cocoa. At last we've found something tasty that we can consume! Pure cocoa is fine as long as - you guessed it! - it does not contain any sugar or sweeteners. It's increasingly being used as a flavour enhancer with people adding it to their coffee and tea and even incorporating it in spices and sauces to accompany meat dishes. More versatile than you might imagine and a welcome guest on the menu!

Carob. Often used as a substitute for chocolate, this legume is usually consumed as carob powder. Happily the powder is made from the pod rather than the potentially harmful seed of the carob. So as long as you avoid the seeds, carob is a good food choice as far as healthy eating is concerned.

Chia. These are another great choice is a healthy eating plan. Chia seeds are not part of the same family of seeds that we find in grains and legumes so they're fine to eat.

Citric Acid. We often find it used as a preservative in canned produce and in jars of preserved foods. Amongst all the harmful substances that are used as food additives, citric acid stands out as one of the few products that is completely acceptable.

Coconut water. It's naturally sweet and delicious but you must check the label to make absolutely sure there is no added sugar. It is not a substitute for fizzy drinks so it's important to limit your consumption. And it isn't a replacement for your daily quota of water. But it is on the goodie list so it's OK to drink and enjoy.

Coffee is good for you. Pure, organic coffee is a potent anti-oxidant and has been linked to a variety of health benefits. Just make sure you don't add sugar, sweeteners, artificial flavourings or milk.

Chocolate is an addictive substance and is the drug of choice for many people. But if you opt for the sugar-free, dairy-free, dark varieties with at least 70% cocoa, you can enjoy your addiction - always in moderation! - with a clear conscience.

Dates contain high quantities of naturally occurring sugar but they are a great source of high octane energy. Feel free to enjoy them but limit your consumption.

Flax seeds are not part of the same group of seeds that are linked to grains, which means that they are a fine source of nutrition.

French fries are a particularly unhealthy way to enjoy potatoes. The problem lies in the fact that they are fried in vegetable oil and this is off limits to anyone seeking to control their weight and boost their wellbeing. If you make your own fries at home, you can use coconut oil instead of vegetable oil or you can bake them or roast them to avoid the frying problem altogether.

Fruit juice is off the agenda. That's right. Fruit juice delivers way too much sugar to your bloodstream way too quickly and produces a massive insulin reaction. Not good! The only way to enjoy fruit juice is when it's still inside the fruit. The body has to work a lot harder to extract the energy from the fruit pulp and this slows down the absorption rate of the sugars, avoiding the sudden sugar rush and the subsequent dramatic fall off as the insulin kicks in. There's an enormous amount of advertising surrounding the supposed health benefits of drinking fruit juice. It's giving you the wrong information. Stick to the fruit instead and live longer.

Guar gum is a natural thickener and it's a perfectly acceptable item on your food list.

Green beans get our yes vote despite the fact that they're a legume and contain seeds. But green beans have very small, immature seeds inside a large green pod so the potential for damage is correspondingly small.

Hemp seeds are a great source of healthy protein. They're not related to the harmful seeds that occur in grains so you're free to add hemp seeds to your diet plan and enjoy the benefits.

Hummus always looks so healthy but it's made from a not so healthy legume, the garbanzo bean or chick pea. It seems tough, but hummus just got fired from the list.

Mayonnaise usually contains sugar. I know. It's everywhere. Even the healthy-sounding olive oil based mayo is largely made up from soybean oil so your best alternative is to make your own. It really is fast and easy. Organic eggs (one yolk) and extra virgin olive oil (one cup), a little apple cider vinegar(2 teaspoons), a pinch of garlic powder and black pepper to taste...and you'll be amazed how great real mayo tastes.

Mustard is a great gift to many meals, adding some much-needed flavour to otherwise bland and tasteless dishes. Just be careful about the label. Some manufacturers add flavourings, sugar, colouring agents and wine. Pure and natural are your watchwords. Once again make your own with a seed grinder, one cup ground (semi) mustard seeds, two tablespoons olive oil, one tablespoon apple cider vinegar and stevia to taste.

Potatoes are a surprising candidate for healthy eating. All varieties get the stamp of approval. If you're conscious of the need to lose weight, be careful with the larger calorie-dense white varieties. You can eat them, of course, but you are much better off with the small red skinned potatoes and you need to eat them sparingly. Needless to say perhaps, but you need to avoid the commercially prepared, deep fried potato chips or French fries.

Anti-Inflammatory Diet Your Pathway to Looking and Feeling 10 Years Younger
By Beran Parry

Protein shakes have become increasingly popular as the protein diet fashion has persuaded countless individuals to use a scoop of protein powder as a substitute for intelligent nutrition. But have you read the ingredients on the label? Protein shakes are full of the things you really need to avoid if you're planning on losing weight and getting seriously healthy. The only exception to the rule is our old friend hemp. Hemp protein powder can be a useful assistant in your health and wellbeing plan because your body works so well with this potent little seed.

Quinoa can be found filling the shelves in health stores everywhere but it can act very much like a grain and produce similarly harmful effects. Quinoa just got cancelled. The same applies to buckwheat, amaranth and other gluten-free grain substitutes.

Safflower or sunflower oil is also off the menu because we want to cut out vegetable oils as much as possible.

Salt is an important part of the human diet. You might not know that iodised table salt also contains a sugar in the form of dextrose. This sugar is used to block the oxidisation process that would effectively neutralise the potassium iodine that's an important part of iodised salt. You still need salt in your diet and it's almost impossible to eat outside of the house without encountering iodised salt: it's added to restaurant and processed food as standard.

Smoothies get top marks for health as long as they're based on fresh vegetables. no colourants, unnatural flavourings or artificial additives.

Stevia is the only sweetener that passes our healthy additive test. It's natural and we recommend the less-processed leaf rather than the liquid or powder versions.

Tahini is made from sesame seeds and gets a welcome 'Yes' on our list of acceptable, healthy foods. Plus it tastes really, really great!

Vanilla extract is such a favourite flavour enhancer in so many baking recipes but it usually contains sugar or alcohol. The extract is a no-no but you can use vanilla bean powder to get the super flavour without the sugar or alcohol additives.

Growing Younger DELICIOUS DINING GUIDE

Whether by choice or profession, you will at some point find yourself at a restaurant, with the challenge of what to eat. Restaurant menus can be a confusing territory – but these tips will make your healthy dining experience fun, satisfying, and stress-free.

Anti-Inflammatory Diet Your Pathway to Looking and Feeling 10 Years Younger
By Beran Parry

Ahead of time

- Call ahead to make sure the restaurant will cope with your requirements.
- When dining with a group, take charge and suggest a restaurant that meets your specifications.
- Smaller, local restaurants are generally more accommodating to substitutions or customization than larger chains.
- Research the menu beforehand and plan your order so you won't be tempted by other less healthy dishes when you arrive.
- Pack your own small bottle of dressing. Don't make a big deal out of it and most servers won't say anything.

When seated

- Upon being seated, ask the server not to serve you bread.
- Don't hesitate to ask about food sourcing, hidden ingredients (like cheese on a salad), or preparation methods.
- Be specific about any allergies, sensitivities, or preferences, especially if you experience health consequences when exposed – write them down for the chef if there is confusion.

Ordering

- Be firm but nice about your requests. Say things like, "Would it be possible…?" or "I'd love it if…"
- Get creative! Order sandwiches without bread, pasta toppings on a bed of spinach, or double vegetables as your side.
- If you've got wild-caught or organic protein options, choose those above conventionally raised protein.
- Ask for vegetables to be steamed or sautéed with olive oil, instead of cooked or fried in vegetable oil.
- Omelets are often infused with milk or pancake batter (!) to make them fluffier. Request boiled eggs, or order them poached.
- Request individual bottles of olive oil and vinegar and some fresh lemon to use as a dressing on salad, vegetables, or protein.

Bill, please

- When you have a good experience, thank the server and the chef – and tip well, especially if the restaurant is one you visit often.

Anti-Inflammatory Diet Your Pathway to Looking and Feeling 10 Years Younger
By Beran Parry

- Relax about being assertive with your demands – you are the customer after all!
- Make it a top priority to never be compromised in a restaurant again!

Anti-Inflammatory Diet Your Pathway to Looking and Feeling 10 Years Younger
By Beran Parry

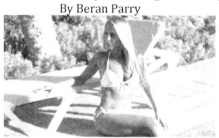

Chapter 16:

FIFTY 10 YEARS YOUNGER Recipes at your disposal

All these delicious recipes are unbelievably tasty and they are ALL:

Grain free

Gluten free

Dairy free

Sugar Free

Processed Free

Low Sodium

The great news is that they are all suitable for everyday use or whenever you want to create mouth wateringly tantalising delights.

Enjoy and to benefit even more consider downloading the Skinny Delicious Recipe Book by pre-ordering it on this link.....

Anti-Inflammatory Diet Your Pathway to Looking and Feeling 10 Years Younger
By Beran Parry

1. Ginger Carrot Protein Smoothie

Ingredients:

3/4 cup carrot juice

1 tablespoon hemp protein powder

1 tablespoon hulled hemp seeds

1/2 apple

3 to 4 ice cubes

1/2 inch piece fresh ginger

Instructions:

Add to a blender and blend until smooth.

2. Raspberry Coconut Smoothie

Ingredients:

½ - 1 cup coconut milk (depending on how thick you like it)

1 medium banana, peeled sliced and frozen

2 teaspoons coconut extract (optional)

1 cup frozen raspberries

1 tablespoon hemp protein powder

Optional: shredded coconut flakes, and stevia to taste

Instructions:

Add coconut milk, frozen banana slices and coconut extract to your blender.

Pulse 1-2 minutes until smooth.

Add frozen raspberries and continue to pulse until smooth.

Pour into your serving glass, top with a couple of raspberries and a little shredded coconut, and enjoy!

3. Pineapple Protein Smoothie

Ingredients:

1 cup (135g) pineapple chunks

1 cup (200g) coconut milk (fresh or tinned)

½ med (65g) banana

¼ cup (65g) ice cubes

¼ tsp vanilla bean powder

Pinch low sodium salt

1 tablespoon hemp protein powder

Instructions:

Peel pineapple and chop into small chunks.

Put everything into a high speed blender and blend until smooth.

4. High Protein and Nutritional Delish Smoothie

Ingredients:

1 cup almond milk

1/2 Avocado

4 Strawberries

1/2 Bananas (Very ripe)

1/2 cup Raw Kale or spinach

1/4 cup Carrot or 100 % Orange Juice (legal) (water can be subbed)

1 cup Coconut Yogurt..or almond milk)

1 tablespoon hemp protein powder

Instructions:

Add everything to your blender, Bullet, Ninja, etc

More water or ice can be added to help with your preferred texture/thickness.

5. Tantalizing Key Lime Pie Smoothie

Ingredients:

1 cup coconut milk

1 cup ice

1/2 avocado

zest and juice of 2 limes

Pure liquid stevia to taste

1 tablespoon hemp protein powder

Instructions:

Add all ingredients to Vitamix or blender and blend until smooth.

Anti-Inflammatory Diet Your Pathway to Looking and Feeling 10 Years Younger
By Beran Parry

SKINNY DELICIOUS
SOUPS

6. Zucchini Fish Soup Delight!

Ingredients:

4 cups chicken broth, I used a low-sodium organic brand

2 cups zucchini noodles made with a spiralizer (2 zucchini)

2-3 cups cooked sliced white fish of choice

2/3 tsp fish sauce

1 1/2 tsp grated fresh ginger

Fresh herbs (handful): basil, mint, cilantro (whichever you prefer)

Sliced scallions, as much as you like

Thin slices of jalapeño

Lime wedges

Thin slices of red onion

Instructions:

In a medium-sized pot, heat the broth on medium heat until it becomes steamy.

Add the ginger (my favourite component!), , fish sauce and about 2 tablespoons of the herbs.

Simmer for a few minutes.

I added my jalapeño slices during this step because I like it spicier, but if you don't like it as spicy, wait until garnishing to add them.

Add your fish, zucchini and cook for about 4 minutes, until your noodles get soft and your meat is warmed.

Serve with the fresh herbs, jalapeño slices, lime wedges, and red onion slices as you like!

7. Roasted Winter Vegetable Turkey Soup

Ingredients:

2 large onions, cut into eighths

2 large sweet potatoes, peeled and cut into 1 inch dice

2 lbs of carrots, peeled and cut into 2 inch dice

1 head (yes head) of garlic, cloves peeled

4 tbsp coconut oil

low sodium salt and pepper to taste

2 cups low sodium chicken stock

1-2 turkey breasts

Instructions:

Preheat the oven to 425 degrees F.

Distribute the onions, garlic, sweet potatoes and carrots evenly on a sheet tray- it will likely require two trays.

Top the vegetables with coconut oil. You can melt the oil ahead of time if it is solid, or wait until it melts in the oven and then stir it around. Season GENEROUSLY with low sodium salt and pepper.

Roast for 25-35 minutes until vegetables are tender, flipping halfway through cooking.

When the veggies have roasted, transfer them into a large pot on the stove top. Add just enough chicken stock to cover the veggies by 1 inch.

Put the lid on and bring the liquid to a boil. Reduce the heat and simmer with the lid cracked for 10 minutes.

Now you get to puree your soup! You can do this in a blender, but do it in small batches so that it doesn't explode on you. But I love to use my immersion blender. It's convenient and you don't have to mess with all of the transferring and what not.

Taste and season with low sodium salt and pepper if needed.

Spoon it up and eat it as is, or stir in a bit of coconut cream add turkey- Enjoy!

8. Turkey Squash Soup

Ingredients:

1 large acorn squash

1/2 teaspoon olive oil

low sodium salt and pepper to taste

2 cups chicken or vegetable stock

1/4 cup coconut milk

1-2 turkey breasts shredded

3/4 teaspoon ground ginger

Pinch or two of cayenne pepper

Pomegranate seeds and/or sliced almonds, for serving

Instructions:

Preheat the oven to 400. Cut the acorn squash in half and scoop out the seeds and pulp. Brush each half with about 1/4 teaspoon olive oil and sprinkle with low sodium salt and pepper. Place in a foil-lined baking pan and roast, cut sides up, until fork tender (about an hour).

When the squash is cool enough to handle, scoop out the flesh and place it in a medium saucepan, or in a blender if you don't have an immersion blender. Add the remaining ingredients and process with an immersion blender (or regular blender) until smooth. Place the saucepan over medium heat and cook, stirring often, until heated through. Serve hot or warm, with pomegranate seeds and/or sliced almonds.

9. Delicious Lemon-Garlic Soup

Option – add 6 shrimps

Ingredients:

1 tablespoon olive oil

1 tablespoon crushed and chopped fresh garlic

6 cups good-quality low sodium shellfish stock (or mushroom or chicken stock)

2 eggs

1/3 to 1/2 cup fresh lemon juice

1 tablespoon coconut flour for thickening

1/4 teaspoon ground white pepper

chopped fresh cilantro or parsley, if desired

Instructions:

In a 4-quart pot, heat the olive oil over medium-high heat and saute the garlic for 1-2 minutes, or until just fragrant. Do not let the garlic brown.

Reserve 1/2 cup of the stock to mix with the eggs. Pour the remaining 5 1/2 cups of stock into the pot with the garlic. Let the mixture come to a simmer.

In a small bowl, whisk together the eggs, lemon juice, arrowroot, white pepper, and half of a cup of reserved stock. Pour the mixture into the simmering stock and stir until it all thickens--this will only take a few minutes.

Serve the soup hot, sprinkled with fresh cilantro or parsley.

10. Creamy Chicken Soup

Ingredients:

1/2 cup coconut oil, olive oil, or other oil of choice

2 stalks celery, finely diced

2 medium carrots, finely diced

6 cups low sodium chicken broth

1/2 cup cool water 1 teaspoon dried parsley

1/2 teaspoon dried thyme

1 bay leaf

2 teaspoons low sodium salt 3 cups cooked chicken, cubed

1 1/2 cups coconut milk (1 can full-fat canned or homemade; or pureed cauliflower; see Notes for alternate version)

Instructions:

Place oil in a large soup pot over medium heat. Add the celery and carrots. Cook, stirring occasionally, until soft, 10 to 15 minutes.

Add broth. If using arrowroot, place it and 1/2 cup cool water in a small bowl or jar and whisk or shake to combine. Add to pot along with parsley, thyme, bay leaf, and low sodium salt. Cook, stirring occasionally, until bubbly and thickened (if using arrowroot).

Reduce heat, just enough to maintain a boil, and cook, stirring occasionally for 15 minutes.

Stir in coconut milk (or pureed cauliflower) and chicken and heat through. This is a fairly thick soup; if you like it thinner, add more water, broth, or coconut milk and heat through. Remove bay leaf just before serving. Leftovers may be frozen.

Note:

Alternatively, you can use pureed cauliflower instead of the coconut milk. This version is just as creamy.

To puree the cauliflower, place florets from two medium heads in a pot. Optionally, add a peeled and smashed garlic clove. Add water to cover and about 1/2 tablespoon low sodium salt. Boil 20 minutes or until soft. Drain away water and puree until very smooth using hand blender or other method. Yield is about 4 cups; add the entire amount to the soup.

11. Creamy Carrot Salad

Ingredients:

1 pound carrots - shredded

20 ounces crushed pineapple -- drained

8 ounces Coconut milk

3/4 cup flaked coconut

Stevia to taste

Shredded turkey one breast

Instructions:

Combine all ingredients, tossing well. Cover and chill.

12. Tasty Carrot Salad

Ingredients:

5 carrots, medium

1 tbs. whole black mustard seeds

1/4 tsp. low sodium salt

2 tsp. lemon juice

2 tbs. olive oil

Add 1 Grated egg on top

Instructions:

Trim and peel and grate carrots. In a bowl, toss with low sodium salt and set aside.

In a small heavy pan over medium heat, heat oil.

When very hot, add mustard seeds. As soon as the seeds begin to pop, in a few seconds, pour oil and seeds over carrots.

Add lemon juice and toss. Serve at room temperature or cold.

Add Grated egg.

13. Asian Aspiration Salad

Ingredients:

1 red bell pepper, sliced

1 large carrot, cut into matchsticks

1 cucumber, halved lengthwise and sliced

Optional:

fresh ginger juice and rice vinegar

2 boiled eggs

Instructions:

Mix ingredients and Serve.

14. Italian Tuna Bonanza Salad

Ingredients:

10 sun-dried tomatoes

2 (5 oz) can of tuna

1-2 ribs of celery, diced finely

2 Tablespoons of extra virgin olive oil

1 cloves garlic, minced

3 Tablespoons finely chopped parsley

1/2 Tablespoon lemon juice

low sodium salt and pepper to taste

Instructions:

Prepare the sun-dried tomatoes by softening them in warm water for 30 minutes until soft. Then, pat the tomatoes dry and chop finely.

Flake the tuna. and mix the tuna together with the chopped tomatoes, celery, extra virgin olive oil, garlic, parsley, and lemon juice. Add low sodium salt and pepper to taste.

If not serving immediately, mix with extra olive oil just before serving.

Optional: Make cucumber boats with them.

15. Incredibly Delish Avocado Tuna Salad

Ingredients:

1 avocado

1 lemon, juiced, to taste

1 tablespoon chopped onion, to taste

5 ounces cooked or canned wild tuna

low sodium salt and pepper to taste

Instructions:

Cut the avocado in half and scoop the middle of both avocado halves into a bowl, leaving a shell of avocado flesh about 1/4-inch thick on each half.

Add lemon juice and onion to the avocado in the bowl and mash together. Add tuna, low sodium salt and pepper, and stir to combine. Taste and adjust if needed.

Fill avocado shells with tuna salad and serve.

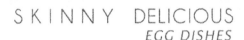

SKINNY DELICIOUS
EGG DISHES

16. Avocado and Shrimp Omelette

Ingredients:

6 eggs

2 Tbsp. chopped parsley

2 Tbsp. lemon juice, divided

1/4 tsp. salt

1/8 tsp. cayenne pepper

1 large* ripe avocado, diced

1 1/2 Tbsp. avocado oil

3 oz. bay shrimp

3 parsley sprigs

Instructions:

Beat together eggs, parsley, 3/4 of the lemon juice, salt, and cayenne pepper; reserve.

Gently toss avocado with remaining lemon juice; reserve.

Heat oil in an omelette pan. (Use a large omelette pan for four or more servings.)

Pour egg mixture into pan.

Cook over medium heat, lifting edges and tilting pan to allow uncooked egg to run under, until set but still moist on top.

Scatter reserved avocado and shrimp over omelette.

Fold omelette in half; heat another minute or two.

Slide onto a warmed serving plate; garnish with parsley sprigs.

To serve, cut omelette into wedges.

Anti-Inflammatory Diet Your Pathway to Looking and Feeling 10 Years Younger
By Beran Parry

17. Mushrooms, Eggs and Onion Bonanza

Ingredients:

1 medium onion, finely diced

1/4 cup coconut oil

10-12 medium white mushrooms, finely chopped

12 hard boiled eggs, peeled and finely chopped

Freshly ground black pepper to taste

Instructions:

Saute the onion in coconut oil until golden brown.

Add the mushrooms and saute another 5 minutes or so, stirring frequently, until mushrooms are softened and turned dark.

Remove from heat and let cool.

Mix together with the eggs and pepper. Chill until ready to serve.

Anti-Inflammatory Diet Your Pathway to Looking and Feeling 10 Years Younger
By Beran Parry

18. Spectacular Eggie Salsa

Ingredients:

2 pounds fresh ripe tomatoes, peeled and coarsely chopped

2 to 3 serrano or jalapeño chillies, seeded for a milder sauce, and chopped

2 garlic cloves, peeled, halved, green shoots removed

1/2 small onion, chopped

2 tablespoons oil

Low sodium salt to taste

4 to 8 eggs (to taste)

Chopped cilantro for garnish

Instructions:

Place the tomatoes, chillies, garlic and onion in a blender and puree, retaining a bit of texture.

Heat 1 tablespoon of the oil over high heat in a large, heavy nonstick skillet, until a drop of puree will sizzle when it hits the pan.

Add the puree and cook, stirring, for four to ten minutes, until the sauce thickens, darkens and leaves a trough when you run a spoon down the middle of the pan. It should just begin to stick to the pan.

Season to taste with salt, and remove from the heat. Keep warm while you fry the eggs.

Warm four plates. Fry the eggs in a heavy skillet over medium-high heat.

Use the remaining tablespoon of oil if necessary. Cook them sunny side up, until the whites are solid but the yolks still runny.

Season with salt and pepper, and turn off the heat. Place one or two fried eggs on each plate.

Spoon the hot salsa over the whites of the eggs, leaving the yolks exposed if possible. Sprinkle with cilantro and serve.

19. Delish Veggie Hash With Eggs

Ingredients:

2 tablespoon extra virgin olive oil

2 garlic cloves, minced

1/4 cup sweet white onion, chopped

1 cup yellow squash, chopped

1/2 cup mushroom, sliced

Low sodium salt and pepper

1 cup cherry tomatoes, halved

1 cup fresh spinach, chopped

4 eggs, poached or cooked any style

You can substitute the squash with whatever vegetables you have

Instructions:

Heat large non-stick skillet over medium heat. Add olive oil to pan.

Add garlic and onion and saute for 2 minutes, then add chopped squash or your favourite vegetable, cook for 2 more minutes, then add mushrooms. Cook for 5-minutes or until almost compete.

At this point add low sodium salt and pepper, then add tomatoes and spinach and cook until spinach wilts. Drain well before plating.

While finishing this prepare eggs to your liking in another pan.

To serve, drained hash mixture to and then add to individual plates. On top of hash add 2 cooked eggs per person.

20. Spicy Spinach Bake

Ingredients:

6 eggs

1 bunch fresh spinach chopped (a box of frozen will do if you do not have fresh)

1/2 tsp hot pepper flakes

Olive oil

Low sodium Salt and pepper

Instructions:

Scramble the eggs in a bowl. Add the spinach, low sodium salt and pepper.

Scramble together. Heat a large non-stick skillet with about 1/2 cup olive oil.

When the oil is hot put the hot pepper flakes in then pour the mixture in. When it starts to cook on the bottom, flip it over.

1. Try not to cook it until it is dry, take it out when it is medium scrambled. Let cool and eat.

21. Zucchini Casserole

Ingredients:

3 large zucchini

1/2 red onion, chopped

1/2 cup mushrooms

5 eggs

1 tsp low sodium salt

Freshly ground black pepper, to taste

Instructions:

Preheat oven to 375 degrees F..

Grate all of the zucchini and put into a large bowl.

In a separate bowl, beat the eggs with low sodium salt and pepper.

Combine all of the ingredients, in the large bowl and mix together. You want to have enough eggs to coat the whole mixture.

Warm about a 1/2 tablespoon of olive oil in the skillet over medium heat.

Add the zucchini mixture into the pan. Cover and cook about 5 minutes until the eggs start to set on the bottom.

Transfer to the oven and bake for 12-15 minutes, until the eggs are firm. Remove and let rest for 5-10 minutes, then serve.

22. Spicy Granola

Ingredients:

1 ½ cups almond flour

1/3 cup coconut oil

2 tsp cinnamon

2 tsp nutmeg

2 tsp vanilla extract

½ cup walnuts

½ cup coconut flakes

¼ cup hemp seeds

low sodium salt, to taste

Instructions:

Preheat oven to 275 degrees Fahrenheit.

Combine all ingredients in a large mixing bowl and mix well. (I find it easier to melt down the coconut oil a little bit before adding it)

Spread mixture into one flat layer on a greased baking sheet.

Bake for 40-50 minutes, or until mixture is toasted to your liking.

Remove from oven and allow to cool before serving, then transfer into a plastic container to save the rest!

23. Breakfast Mexicana

Ingredients:

For the tortillas:

2 eggs

2 egg whites

1/2 cup water

4 tsp ground flaxseed

Pinch of low sodium salt

For the filling:

1 avocado, diced

1/4 cup red bell

pepper, finely diced

1/4 cup onion, finely diced

1/4 cup baked cod or other protein

Handful of spinach leaves

1 tsp coconut oil

Instructions:

In a small bowl, whisk together the ingredients for the tortilla. Preheat the oven

Heat a 10-inch non-stick skillet over medium heat and coat well with coconut oil spray.

Pour half of the tortilla mixture into the pan and swirl to evenly distribute.

Using a metal spatula, loosen the edges of the tortilla from the pan.

Cook a couple of minutes until golden brown on the bottom, and then carefully slide the spatula under the tortilla to loosen it from the bottom of the pan. Do not flip yet.

Place the pan under the broiler for 3-4 minutes until the tortilla gets a little bubbly.

Remove the tortilla from the pan, setting on a piece of aluminium foil. Repeat with other half of tortilla mixture.

After the tortillas are done broiling, preheat the oven to 400 degrees F. In a separate small pan, heat the coconut oil over medium heat.

Add the onions and peppers and sauté for 5-8 minutes, until soft. Add the spinach into the pan and wilt.

Place all of the fillings down the center of the tortillas and wrap tightly. Place into the oven for 5-8 minutes to set. It's so delish!

24. Gutsy Granola

Ingredients:

1 cup cashews

3/4 cup almonds

1/4 cup pumpkin seeds, shelled

1/4 cup sunflower seeds, shelled

1/2 cup unsweetened coconut flakes

1/4 cup coconut oil

Stevia to taste

1 tsp vanilla

1 tsp low sodium salt

Instructions:

Preheat oven to 300 degrees F. Line a baking sheet with parchment paper. Place the cashews, almonds, coconut flakes and pumpkin seeds into a blender and pulse to break the mixture into smaller pieces.

In a large microwave-safe bowl, melt the coconut oil, vanilla, and honey together for 40-50 seconds. Add in the mixture from the blender and the sunflower seeds, and stir to coat.

Spread the mixture out onto the baking sheet and cook for 20-25 minutes, stirring once, until the mixture is lightly browned. Remove from heat. Add low sodium salt.

Press the granola mixture together to form a flat, even surface. Cool for about 15 minutes, and then break into chunks.

25. Delish Veggie Breakfast Peppers

Ingredients:

2 bell peppers – your choice of colour

4 eggs

1 cup white mushrooms

1 cup broccoli

¼ tsp cayenne pepper

low sodium salt and pepper, to taste

Instructions:

Preheat oven to 375 degrees Fahrenheit.

Dice up your vegetables of choice.

In a medium sized bowl, mix eggs, low sodium salt, pepper, cayenne pepper, and vegetables.

Cut peppers into equal halves. A tip:

Core the peppers so that they're clean enough to add the filling.

Pour a quarter of the egg / vegetable mix into each pepper halve, adding more vegetables to the top to fill in any empty space.

Place on baking sheet and cook approximately 35 minutes.

Anti-Inflammatory Diet Your Pathway to Looking and Feeling 10 Years Younger
By Beran Parry

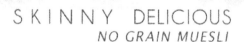

SKINNY DELICIOUS
NO GRAIN MUESLI

26. Tasty Apple Almond Coconut Medley

Ingredients:

one-half apple cored and roughly diced

handful of sliced almonds

handful of unsweetened coconut

generous dose of cinnamon

1 pinch of low sodium salt

Instructions:

Pulse in the food processor to desired consistency—smaller is better for the little ones! Serve with almond milk, or creamy coconut milk.

27. Sweetie Skinny Crackers

Ingredients:

1 egg

2 tablespoons pure liquid stevia

1 Tbspn coconut oil, melted

1.5 cups almond flour

.5 cup coconut flour

1 teaspoon cinnamon

Instructions:

Preheat oven to 350°

In a large bowl, whisk together the egg, pure liquid stevia and melted coconut oil

Add the coconut and almond flour and stir to combine.

Give the dough a couple of kneads so it's well incorporated

Turn the dough onto a piece of parchment paper and flatten a bit with your hands.

Place another piece of parchment on top and roll out with a rolling pin until it's about 1/8 inch thick.

Remove the top piece of parchment and cut the dough into 1/4 inch squares for cereal, and about 2"x3" for crackers

Sprinkle the cinnamon into the dough mixture.

Slide the dough with the bottom parchment paper onto a baking sheet and bake for 15 minutes.

Turn down the oven to 325° and bake for another 10-15 minutes, or until the cereal / crackers are crisp.

28. Apple Chia Delight

Ingredients:

2c organic chia seeds (black or white)

1c organic hemp hearts

1/2 chopped dried organic apples (or other dried fruit of your choice)

2tbsp real cinnamon

1 tsp low sodium salt

optional: 1/2c chopped nuts of your choice

Instructions:

Throw all of this together, mix it up, and store in a jar in a cool dry place. Stevia to taste.

29. Ultimate Skinny Granola

Ingredients:

1 cup of unsweetened coconut milk or unsweetened almond milk or kefir

Stevia liquid to taste

1 tspoon of unsalted pecan pieces

1 tspoon of unsalted walnut pieces

1 tspoon of silvered almonds

1 tspoon of unsalted pistachios

1 tspoon of unsalted raw pine nuts

1 tspoon of unsalted, raw sunflower/safflower seeds

1 tspoon of unsalted, raw pumpkin seeds

2 Tbspoons of frozen or fresh berry selection (e.g. blueberries, blackberries, raspberries, strawberries, or other kinds etc)

Instructions:

Put all the nuts & seeds in a breakfast bowl.

If using unsweetened milk, you could optionally add a teaspoon of pure liquid stevia and stir it well in.

Add the berries and milk.

If using frozen berries, wait for 2-3 minutes for them to get warmer.

The berries will now release some colour into the milk, making it look really interesting. Enjoy!

30. Divine Protein Muesli

Ingredients:

1 cup unsweetened unsulfured coconut flakes

1 tbsp chopped walnuts

1 tbsp raw almonds (~10)

1 tbsp chocolate chips (soy, dairy, and gluten free brand)

1/2 tsp cinnamon (Ceylon)

1 cup unsweetened almond milk

1 scoop hemp protein

Instructions:

In a medium bowl layer coconut flakes, walnuts, almonds, raisins and chocolate chips.

Sprinkle with cinnamon.

Pour cold almond milk over the muesli and eat with a spoon.

Anti-Inflammatory Diet Your Pathway to Looking and Feeling 10 Years Younger
By Beran Parry

SKINNY DELICIOUS
MAIN COURSES

31. Prawn garlic Fried "Rice"

Ingredients:

1 tbsp coconut oil

1 cup white onion, finely chopped

2 cloves garlic, minced

8 oz. prawns peeled and deveined

1 medium carrot, chopped

1/2 cup peas

2 cups cooked cauliflower rice

2 eggs, beaten

Low sodium salt and pepper, to taste

Instructions:

Heat a wok or large pan over medium-high heat. Melt the coconut oil and add the onion and garlic to the pan.

Cook for 3-4 minutes until the onion starts to soften. Add the shrimp and cook for 1 minute.

Add the carrot, peas, and bell pepper to the pan. Cook for 3-4 minutes, and then stir in the cauliflower rice.

Clear a circle in the center of the pan and pour in the beaten eggs. Stir to scramble the eggs and then combine with the other ingredients.

Season with low sodium salt and pepper to taste.

32. Delish Baked dill Salmon

Ingredients:

2 6-oz. salmon fillets

2 zucchini, halved lengthwise and thinly sliced

1/4 red onion, thinly sliced

1 tsp fresh dill, chopped

2 slices lemon

1 tbsp fresh lemon juice

Extra virgin olive oil, for drizzling

low sodium salt and freshly

ground pepper

Instructions:

Preheat the oven to 350 degrees F. Prepare a baking tray

Place half of the zucchini, red onion, dill, and one lemon slice. Drizzle with olive oil and sprinkle with low sodium salt and pepper. Place a salmon fillet on top and drizzle with the lemon juice. Season with low sodium salt and pepper. Repeat with the remaining ingredients.

Bake for 15-20 minutes until the salmon is opaque.

33. Ostrich Steak or Venison with Divine Mustard Sauce and Roasted Tomatoes

Ingredients:

For the tomatoes:

2 pints cherry tomatoes, halved

2 tbsp extra virgin olive oil

Stevia to taste

low sodium salt and freshly ground pepper

For the cauliflower rice:

1/2 head of cauliflower, chopped coarsely

1/2 small onion, finely diced

1 tbsp coconut oil

1 tbsp fresh parsley, chopped

low sodium salt and freshly ground pepper, to taste

For the meat:

4 Ostrich or venison steaks

Extra virgin olive oil

low sodium salt and freshly ground pepper

Coconut oil, for the pan

For the sauce:

Anti-Inflammatory Diet Your Pathway to Looking and Feeling 10 Years Younger
By Beran Parry

1/4 cup red onion, finely diced

1/4 cup apple cider vinegar

1 cup low sodium chicken stock

1 tbsp whole grain mustard

low sodium salt and freshly ground pepper, to taste

Instructions:

Preheat the oven to 400 degrees F. Place the tomatoes on a baking sheet and drizzle with olive oil and honey. Sprinkle with low sodium salt and pepper and toss to coat evenly. Bake for 15-20 minutes until soft.

While the tomatoes are roasting, prepare the cauliflower rice. Place the cauliflower into a food processor and pulse until reduced to the size of rice grains.

Melt the coconut oil in a nonstick skillet over medium heat. Add the onion and cook for 5-6 minutes until translucent. Stir in the cauliflower, season with low sodium salt and pepper, and cover. Cook for 7-10 minutes until the cauliflower has softened, and then toss with parsley.

To make the lamb, preheat the oven to 325 degrees F. Pat the ostrich or venison dry and rub with olive oil. Generously season both sides with low sodium salt and pepper.

Heat one tablespoon of coconut oil in a cast iron skillet. When the pan is hot, add to the pan and sear for 2-3 minutes on all sides until golden brown.

Place the skillet in the oven and bake for 5-8 minutes until the ostrich or venison reaches desired doneness. Let rest for 10 minutes before serving.

While the meat is resting, add the red onion to the skillet with the pan drippings from the lamb. Sauté for 3-4 minutes, then add the white wine vinegar.

Turn the heat to high and cook until the vinegar has mostly evaporated. Add the stock and bring to a boil, cooking until the sauce reduces by half.

Stir in the mustard, and season to taste with low sodium salt and pepper. Pour over ostrich or venison to serve.

34. Scrumptious Cod in Delish Sauce

Ingredients:

1 lb. cod fillets

1/3 cup almond flour

1/2 tsp low sodium salt

2-3 tbsp extra virgin olive oil

2 tbsp walnut oil, divided

3/4 cup low sodium chicken stock

3 tbsp lemon juice

1/4 cup capers, drained

2 tbsp fresh parsley, chopped

Instructions:

Stir the almond flour and low sodium salt together in a shallow bowl. Rinse off the fish and pat dry with a paper towel. Dredge the fish in the almond flour mixture to coat.

Heat enough olive oil to coat the bottom of a large skillet over medium-high heat along with one tablespoon walnut oil. Working in batches, add the cod and cook for 2-3 minutes per side to brown. Remove to a plate and set aside.

Add the chicken stock, lemon juice, and capers to the same skillet and scrape any browned bits off the bottom. Simmer to reduce the sauce by almost half. Remove from heat and stir in the remaining tablespoon of walnut oil.

To serve, divide the cod onto plates, drizzle with the sauce, and sprinkle with parsley.

35. Delicious Turkey Veggie Lasagne

Ingredients:

For the meat sauce:

1 large yellow onion, coarsely chopped

2 cloves garlic, coarsely chopped

2 tbsp extra virgin olive oil

1 1/2 lbs. ground turkey

1/2 cup tomato paste

1/2 cup tomato sauce

1 cup red wine

1 bay leaf

3 sprigs thyme

low sodium salt and freshly ground pepper, to taste

For the lasagne:

1 eggplant, sliced lengthwise thinly

1 tsp low sodium salt

1 tbsp extra virgin olive oil

2 yellow squash, sliced thinly

1/2 cup torn fresh basil leaves

8 oz. white mushrooms, sliced

Anti-Inflammatory Diet Your Pathway to Looking and Feeling 10 Years Younger By Beran Parry

2 cups fresh spinach

2 large zucchini, sliced lengthwise into ribbons

For the topping:

1/2 head cauliflower

1 tbsp olive oil

1/2 tsp garlic powder

1/2 tsp low sodium salt

Freshly ground pepper, to taste

Instructions:

To make the meat sauce, place the onion and garlic in a food processor and pulse to finely chop.

Heat the olive oil in a heavy-bottomed saucepan over medium heat. Add the onion and garlic and season with low sodium salt and pepper. Cook for 12-15 minutes until beginning to brown, stirring frequently.

Add the turkey to the pot and season with low sodium salt and pepper.

Cook for 15 minutes until browned. Stir in the tomato paste and cook for 2-3 minutes. Add the red wine to the pan and cook for 5 more minutes.

Add the tomato sauce, bay leaf, and thyme to the pan. Bring to a simmer, and then add 1/2 cup water.

Cook at a low simmer for 1 hour, stirring occasionally and adding more water if necessary. Adjust seasonings to taste. Discard the bay leaf and thyme.

Preheat the oven to 350 degrees F. Sprinkle the eggplant with low sodium salt and set aside for 15 minutes to drain. Rinse and pat dry.

Heat one tablespoon of olive oil in a skillet over medium heat. Cook the eggplant for 2-3 minutes per side until golden.

Anti-Inflammatory Diet Your Pathway to Looking and Feeling 10 Years Younger
By Beran Parry

Layer the lasagne in a baking dish. Start by layering the yellow squash as the base. Add one third of the meat sauce on top of that, then lay the eggplant slices, fresh basil, and mushrooms.

Next add the rest of the meat sauce, then the spinach, zucchini, and finally drizzle with olive oil and sprinkle with low sodium salt and pepper. Bake for 40-45 minutes.

While the lasagne is baking, place the cauliflower in a blender and process until it reaches a rice-like consistency.

Add to a skillet and sauté with the olive oil, garlic powder, low sodium salt, and pepper over medium heat.

Cook for 6-8 minutes until soft, adding a tablespoon of water if necessary. After the lasagne has cooked for 20 minutes, sprinkle with the cauliflower and return to the oven for the remaining cooking time. Serve hot.

Anti-Inflammatory Diet Your Pathway to Looking and Feeling 10 Years Younger
By Beran Parry

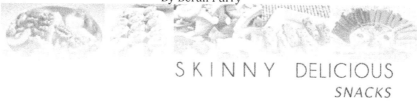

SKINNY DELICIOUS SNACKS

36. Skinny Veggie Dip

Ingredients:

1 tbsp olive oil

1 tsp lemon juice

1 Tbs fresh minced parsley

1 Tbs French minced chives or scallion greens

1 tsp dried dill

1/8 tsp garlic powder

Pinch paprika

low sodium salt and pepper to taste

Instructions:

Combine in triple portions in blender and store to use any time.

37. Delish Cashew Butter Treats

Ingredients:

1 Cup Cashews

Half cup coconut flour

0.5 Cup Cashew Butter

Instructions:

Add the cashews and cashew butter and process until the mixture forms a dough ball.

Add coconut flour to harden the mixture. You may need to scrape down the sides and help the mixture along to form a dough ball.

Once a dough ball has formed, move the dough to a plate to ensure there are no accidents with the food processor blade.

Form the mixture into 16 equal sized balls, refrigerate for at least an hour to harden and enjoy!

38. Chocolate Goji Skinny Bars

Ingredients:

1 cup raw cashews

1/2 cup cocoa powder

1/2 cup dried goji berries

1/2 cup hemp seeds

1 cup shredded coconut

2-3 tbsp coconut oil

2 tbsp liquid stevia

Instructions:

Process cashews in a food processor until it turns into a paste. Roasted cashews don't work as well because they are less sticky.

Transfer paste into a large mixing bowl. Put coconut oil and liquid stevia into another smaller bowl and warm in the oven until it is fully melted.

While this is heating up, add the dried coconut, cocoa powder, and goji berries to the mixing bowl

Transfer melted coconut oil and liquid stevia into mixing bowl.

Everything should now be in the mixing bowl except for the hemp seeds. Mix everything in the bowl with a fork or your hands until thoroughly combined.

This should make a fairly mould-able dough. Spread the hemp seeds onto a plate. Begin to form your dough into small bite-sized balls and then roll them in the hemp seeds until they are thoroughly coated.

Pop in the fridge for at least 2 hours to harden them up a bit.

39. Skinny Power Balls

Ingredients:

1 medium size cooked sweet potato

2 cups almond meal

1 tsp vanilla powder

3 tsp baking powder

3 egg yolks

4 Tbsp melted Coconut Oil

1-2 tsp liquid stevia (I used Sprouts liquid stevia)

3 Tbsp coconut flour (I used Coconut Secret brand)

1 cup of unsweetened shredded coconut and coconut flakes

Instructions:

Peel and mash cooked sweet potato until no more chunks left.

Mix in almond meal, vanilla powder, baking powder until everything incorporates.

Mix in the wet ingredients (egg yolks, melted coconut oil and liquid stevia), stir until everything combines.

Add 3 Tbsp coconut flour. Notice the mixture will be less wet but not too dry. Do not try to put too much coconut flour as it absorbs a lot of moisture and the balls would be too dry and flaky.

Line a baking sheet with a parchment paper. Pre-heat the oven for 350°F

Shape the balls into ping-pong ball size and roll each of them in the bowl of unsweetened shredded coconut and coconut flakes.

Anti-Inflammatory Diet Your Pathway to Looking and Feeling 10 Years Younger
By Beran Parry

Bake the balls in 350°F for about 25 minutes or until the edges turned golden brown or they are dried out already. Remove from heat and let them cool down. The balls are soft when they're still warm but as they cooled down, they should be more firm. After they cooled down, put them in a fridge so they'll be more firm.

40. Butternut Squash-raw Veggie Dip

Ingredients:

1 cup cooked and peeled squash

½ cup COCONUT cream

½ teaspoon low sodium salt

1 teaspoon chipotle paste

1 teaspoon olive oil

1 ½ teaspoons finely chopped shallot

2 teaspoons fresh thyme

¼ teaspoon ground cinnamon

1 teaspoon chili powder

Instructions:

Place squash in a medium bowl and smash with a fork. Add remaining ingredients, mixing until thoroughly combined.

Serve dip with carrot sticks, veggies, or SKINNY CHIPS.

Anti-Inflammatory Diet Your Pathway to Looking and Feeling 10 Years Younger
By Beran Parry

Chapter 17:

The Growing Young Disgracefully Vision

We've covered some very important ground so far in identifying the best ways to get you to the healthier, leaner, ageless new you. Epigenetics prove in the clearest possible terms that we can influence and control our bodies at every level by taking control of what we eat and how we behave.

We've introduced you to the key points in your action plan for wellbeing, emotional health and weight loss control and opened up a whole new world of health and wellbeing possibilities. But we have another important insight to share with you. And now is the perfect moment to reveal it!

Humans have a secret weapon in their behavioural armoury that can work powerfully to help us - or it can work just as powerfully against us. It's our imagination. Or rather it's our ability to visualise. Most of the time, our thoughts drift around in a random pattern of uncoordinated ideas, prompted by whatever happens to pop up around us. We are drawn to whatever grabs our fickle attention.

Our thoughts and feelings are largely conditioned from early childhood experiences that shape our future emotional framework. We learn from an early age to let our thoughts pretty much wander wherever they choose. The mind follows random currents, blown around like a leaf in the wind, lacking focus or any sense of direction. A ship without a rudder.

This is where the risks of self-sabotage emerge; uncontrolled thoughts and feelings, self-doubt, memories of failure, feelings of a lack of self-worth. The list is endless and potentially destructive to our plans for absolute wellbeing. So now is the perfect time to switch on our powers of visualisation and give the mind some clear directions to follow for the future. It's time to bring on the really powerful support system that is hidden within your own mind!

It's incredible to realise how much our expectations shape our perceptions and our behaviour. Our programmed attitudes and responses play a major role in determining many of the outcomes in our lives. Happily, humans possess the immensely powerful gift of visualisation.

By visualising a desired outcome, our behaviours shift to favour those clearly visualised results. The technique of visualisation is incredibly simple. All we have to do is relax. That's right. Relax. Sit down and relax and close your eyes. Now breathe a little more deeply. And see yourself exactly as you really, deeply desire yourself to be.

See your smiling face, see each part of your radiantly healthy, leaner new body. Smile at the strength, health, energy and vitality that surges through your newly visualised body. And feel really

Anti-Inflammatory Diet Your Pathway to Looking and Feeling 10 Years Younger
By Beran Parry

happy about it. Underline the vision with a warm, happy feeling of complete wellbeing. Hold the picture and imagine taking a photograph with your mind. Hear the camera shutter click as you record the stunning new picture of how you are. The picture of who you are becoming.

The powerful vision of the happier, fitter, skinnier new you! Lock this picture in your mind. Hold it in your heart. See it every time you close your eyes. This vision is the future. Use it all the time and you will rally all your hidden creative resources to bring this beautiful new vision of yourself into being.

We do not live in a culture that highlights the importance of mindfulness. We are constantly bombarded by images, noises, distractions and background chaos. We also have to live with the judgement of everyone around us. No wonder we find it difficult to concentrate and to relax. But there are many, simple and effective methods that can help us train our minds to follow our directions and meditation probably offers the simplest, most obvious and direct advantages. There is no religious or philosophical aspect to this exercise. It's just a technique for calming the mind. It takes only fifteen minutes. But it's a method that requires fifteen minutes every day. The daily repetition amplifies the results.

The only equipment you need is a chair, preferably a firm chair with good support for your back. A straight back is supposed to be better for meditation. Being comfortable is also very helpful. Relax your hands on your lap, close your eyes, focus on the spot between your eyebrows and breathe. Just follow your breath gently in and out. That's it. No chanting, humming or repeating strange mantras.

Just good old-fashioned breathing and the focus of concentrating lightly on the breath. The effects are cumulative. They build up gradually as you practise every day. You'll feel calmer. You'll find your powers of concentration improve. You'll be able to relax more easily. Your power to visualise will become more sharply defined. Your mind will begin to follow your directions. You will get a sense of the potential within you. Mastering the mind is a method for mastering ourselves. All this from just fifteen minutes a day. The effects might surprise you because as you learn to become calmer, your body will feel much more comfortable. No prescriptions are required. Just those simple fifteen minutes of daily meditation and you'll soon be looking forward to the sessions with real enthusiasm. You might enjoy the benefits so much that you'll want to meditate for longer.

Your vision of the happier, fitter, leaner new you is the new background picture of your life. It represents the possibility of achieving everything you have chosen for yourself. Every day, you are living the journey of moving towards that possibility. The vision does not have a deadline. There can be no disappointment with the results because you are living every day in the possibility of its realisation.

Even if you slip and go backwards, the vision will put you back on track, guiding you every day towards its fulfillment. That's a powerful tool to have at your disposal. Put it to work right now. Use it

Anti-Inflammatory Diet Your Pathway to Looking and Feeling 10 Years Younger
By Beran Parry

every day. Use it every time you close your eyes and see the vision of how you are transforming yourself.

Ultimately, it's our behaviour that will guide our choices. Meditation is rightly considered to be a very powerful technique for bringing gentle control into the chaos of our minds. As we become more aware of our choices, as we experience the benefits of mindfulness, we can detect old patterns of behaviour that no longer fit our vision of health and vitality. We can understand the advantages of better choices.

We begin to respect the body's needs from a deeper, more caring perspective. The vision represents who we are becoming. The daily meditation helps us to become calmer, more resistant to stress and this healthier emotional framework lends itself to a physically healthier body. We also recommend a short meditation before you go to sleep at night. It's another effective way to calm the mind, still the thoughts and prepare for truly restful sleep.

Meditation has been practised as a tool for managing and directing the mind for thousands of years. It's so effective because we've been using it and refining the techniques as a species for millennia. We've highlighted the fundamental method here because we already use a form of meditation all the time. Have you noticed how easy it can be to day-dream? To drift off into another world of memories or fantasies, oblivious of what's happening around you? A brief reverie or a moment when you lose focus on what's going on around you?

These are altered states of consciousness and they happen all the time. Our purpose with the super simple meditation method is to control that tendency and direct it towards a focused, positive outcome. A way to become mindful yet relaxed. Aware yet calm. Centered yet connected. Still but alive with nurturing, positive energy. And all from fifteen minutes a day! Sounds like the bargain of a lifetime and it's all yours. For now and for the rest of your life.

You've heard it before and you're about to hear it again. We Are What We Eat. There's no getting away from it. You've learned enough by now to understand the vital connection between what you eat and how your body looks. Putting garbage into your body will ruin it. Eat garbage and you'll look like sh.., I mean, waste products. But you know this. That's why you've joined us on this mission of personal transformation.

So far we've been exploring the mechanics of healthy weight control, shedding unwanted pounds and promoting the best health we can possibly enjoy and we fully appreciate the importance of intelligent nutrition. But there are other challenges out there and we've hinted at some of them earlier in Chapter..... We're talking toxins, my friend. Those totally unfriendly substances that pollute our food, poison our drinks and surround us in the air we breathe. Our world has become a scarily toxic place to exist and most of the problems are man-made. That doesn't make them any easier to live with.

Anti-Inflammatory Diet Your Pathway to Looking and Feeling 10 Years Younger
By Beran Parry

You already know how important it is to avoid toxins by eating as naturally as possible but what about the toxins we inhale? What about the poisons that leach into our skin from the environment? The answer to this problem and the best the way to give your body a fair chance to neutralise these poisons is to use a cleansing diet for a few days. Fresh vegetables are the easiest and best source of natural cleansing. They promote natural digestion and contain nutrients that are very helpful in maintaining your health and wellbeing.

Stick to a detox section of the skinny delicious diet for a few days and you'll be amazed at the difference you'll feel in your overall wellness. And drink plenty of water too. The idea of cleansing the body is hardly new. We're just too busy to think of it. But now that we're on a journey of total physical transformation, let's give our bodies the best chance to feel fantastic.

And that means flushing out the garbage to restore total health and wellbeing. Getting away to a place with fresh air is another helpful way to restore balance to your body. Just breathing - and meditating - in the fresh air can work wonders for our health and vitality. Sea air, mountain air, the fresh air in the forest or open countryside can restore you at so many levels. If it's at all possible, make a regular date for a mini cleanse and for some valuable down time in the fresh, open air.

Get a little help from your friends.

You're not alone. It's all too easy to imagine that we're the only ones who are experiencing problems, and think that the rest of the world is having fun, eating well and enjoying life to the full. But most of the world just isn't like that. Sharing your experiences, your challenges and difficulties, sharing your goals and intentions can gather support from everyone around you. You'll be surprised how many people will offer their encouragement and enthusiasm for your new way of life. It will help to reinforce your personal commitment to a healthier, fitter and happier way of being. So feel free to share and build that beautiful support group.

Anti-Inflammatory Diet Your Pathway to Looking and Feeling 10 Years Younger
By Beran Parry

Personal Vision - Summary

Engaging the power of visualisation

Meditating on the powerful new you

Building a clear picture of who you are becoming

Daring to dream and engaging the power of focused visualisation

Total health and well being

Anti-Inflammatory Diet Your Pathway to Looking and Feeling 10 Years Younger
By Beran Parry

Before You Go.......

I am so delighted that you have chosen this book and it's been a pleasure writing it for you. My mission is to help as many readers as possible to benefit from the content you have just been reading. So many of us are able to take new information and apply it to our lives with really positive and long lasting consequences and it is my wish that you have been able to take value from the information I have presented.

Thank you for staying with me during this book and for reading it through to the end. I really hope that you have enjoyed the contents and that's why I appreciate your feedback so much. If you could take a couple of minutes to review the book, your views will help me to create more material that you find beneficial.

I am always thrilled to hear from my readers and you can email me personally at beranparry@gmail.com if you have any questions about this book or future books. Let us know how we can help you by sending a message to the same email address.

Thanks again for your support and encouragement. I really look forward to reading your review.

Stay Healthy!

Anti-Inflammatory Diet Your Pathway to Looking and Feeling 10 Years Younger
By Beran Parry

FOR MORE FROM BERAN PARRY

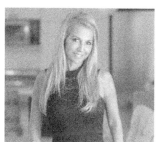

Please search this page over the internet
https://beranparry.com/

Anti-Inflammatory Diet Your Pathway to Looking and Feeling 10 Years Younger
By Beran Parry

Anti-Inflammatory Diet Your Pathway to Looking and Feeling 10 Years Younger
By Beran Parry

As a special seasonal gift I would like to offer you my 5 day Paleo Detox at a 50% discount to do before or after the Holiday Season. It contains the following exciting elements

Delicious Recipes,

Stunning Detox Menu's,

Detoxifying Pilates Exercise Videos,

A Daily Detox Face Pilates Program,

Guided Detox Meditations,

FREE Bonus Recipe Books,

FREE Stress Release System

Here is more info and the coupon code

beranparry.com/midlife-fatburn-detox

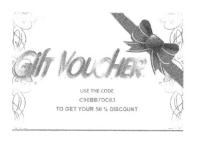

Anti-Inflammatory Diet Your Pathway to Looking and Feeling 10 Years Younger
By Beran Parry

Bibliography

Eating Disorders and the Brain by Bryan Lask

The Paleo Diet Revised: by Dr Loren Cordain PhD

The Protein Boost Diet by Dr Ridha Arem

Eating Well: How to build good eating habits to have your perfect body and overcome eating disorder

Stephen Ecker

The Anderson Method: The Secret to Permanent Weight Loss

William Anderson, Dr. Mark Lupo

The Vitamin D Solution: A 3-Step Strategy to Cure Our Most Common Health Problems

Michael F. Holick Ph.D. M.D., Andrew Weil

OBESITY GENES and their Epigenetic Modifiers by James Baird

Genes and Obesity (Progress in Molecular Biology & Translational Science) by C. Bouchard

Practical Manual of Clinical Obesity by Robert Kushner and Victor Lawrence

The Epigenetics Revolution: How Modern Biology Is Rewriting Our Understanding of Genetics, Disease, and Inheritance...by Nessa Carey

Transgenerational Epigenetics by Trygve Tollefsbol

The Evolution of Obesity by Michael L. Power and Jay Schulkin

The China Study: by Thomas Campbell and T. Colin Campbell

Death by food pyramid by Denise Minger

Primal blueprint by Mark Sissons

Anti-Inflammatory Diet Your Pathway to Looking and Feeling 10 Years Younger
By Beran Parry

The magnesium miracle Dr Carolyn Deane

What are you hungry for by deepak chopra

Gut and Psychology Syndrome: by Dr Natasha Campbell-McBride

Anasti, J. N., H. B. Leonetti, and K. J. Wilson. 2001. Topical progesterone cream has antiproliferative effect on estrogen-stimulated endommetrium. *Obstetrics and Gynecology* (4 Suppl 1): S10.

Leonnetti, H. B., S. Long, and J. N. Anasti. 1999. Transdermal progesterone cream for vasomotor symptoms and postmenopausal bone loss. *Obstetrics and Gynecology* 94:225-28.

Stoll, W. 1987. Phytopharmacon influences atrophic vaginal epithelium: Double-blind study-Cimicifuga vs. estrogenic substances. *Therapeutikon* 1:2-30.

Stolze, H. 1982. An alternative to treat menopausal complaints. *Gyne* 2:4-16.

Kiatz, Ronald and Goldman Robert, The Official Anti-Aging Revolution: Stop the Clock, Time is on Your Side for a Younger, Stronger, Happier You. Dec. 20, 2007

Guabetti, John, Anti-Aging Wisdom – Secrets to Look Younger, Live Longer, and Feel Healthy, Without a Doctor, June 19, 2015

Gifford, Bill, Spring Chicken: Stay Young Forever (or Die Trying), Feb. 17, 2015

White, Miranda E., Aging Backwards: Reverse the Aging Process and Look 10 Years Younger in 30 Minutes a Day, Nov. 11, 2014.

Goldsmith, Theodore, New Truth to the Fountain of Youth: The Emerging Reality of Anti-Aging Medicine, May 4, 2014.

Jacobs, Susan, Anti Aging: How To Look Younger – 7 Easy Steps to Look at Least 10 Years Younger, Jul 24, 2015

Lancer, Harold, Younger: The Breakthrough Anti-Aging Method for Radiant Skin, Feb 4, 2014

Kimball, Maximilian, Healthy Aging: The Mediterranean Diet and Six Great Supplements for Anyone Over 50, Aug 8, 2015

Anti-Inflammatory Diet Your Pathway to Looking and Feeling 10 Years Younger
By Beran Parry

Preston, Carl, Anti-Aging: Superfoods Diet: Lose Weight Naturally, Have Younger Skin and Increase you Energy, Feb 28. 2015

Brooks, Sarah, Natural Cures: 20 Natural Cures, Herbal Medicines, And Natural Remedies For Increased Overall Health And Beauty, Jan 9, 2015

MacGregor, Glynis, Anti-Aging: The Best Beauty Products, Anti Aging Medicines and Skin Care Treatments, Nov 29, 2014

M.D. Weil, Andrew, Healthy Aging: A Lifelong Guide to Your Well-Being, Jan 2, 2007

Made in the USA
Coppell, TX
13 March 2022